WHAT CHRONIC ILLNESS TAUGHT ME

—— Roger Knowles ——

CARGER BOOKS

cargerbooks@gmail.com

Copyright © Roger Knowles 2019

All rights reserved. No part of this publication may be reproduced, stored in a retrieval system, or transmitted in any form or by means, electronic, mechanical, photocopying, recording, or otherwise, without the prior permission of the publisher.

The information contained in this book is for educational purposes only. It is the result of the author's personal research. Whilst the information offered is believed by the author to be true and accurate at the time of going to press, neither the author or publisher can accept any legal responsibility or liability for any errors or omissions that may have been made, or for any adverse effects that may occur as a result of following any recommendations given herein. The author has stressed that he is not a doctor and that he has no medical training of any sort. Always consult a qualified medical practitioner if you have any concerns regarding your health.

ISBN: 9781081713195

OTHER BOOKS BY ROGER KNOWLES

BUG

Broken Cats and Cowboy Hats

Day of Reckoning

The Naked Emperor

To Be a Man

The Association

Dedication

To my wife and soulmate, Hazel, whose journey was as long and tortuous as mine, and who supported me without complaint for the duration. Thank you, Haze, I love you – always have, always will.

Special thanks to….

Carole Glasson, my long time friend and Carger Books partner, without whose tremendous amount of help with this book, it wouldn't exist.

Table of Contents

Introduction vii
Part One – Preliminary Considerations 1
    Chapter One: Desire 2
    Chapter Two: Kiss Frogs 7
    Chapter Three: Beware Of Your Label 9
    Chapter Four: Take Responsibility 12
    Chapter Five: Intuition 14
    Chapter Six: Glimpses 17
    Chapter Seven: Smile 20
    Chapter Eight: Distraction 23
    Chapter Nine: Doctor Knows Best… Sometimes 27
Part Two – Physical considerations 35
    Chapter Ten: Digestion 36
    Chapter Eleven: Diet 50
    Chapter Twelve: Water… What We Drink Matters 62
    Chapter Thirteen: Two Simple Routes To Super Nutrition 69
    Chapter Fourteen: What I Have For Breakfast And Why 75
    Chapter Fifteen: Supplements 85
    Chapter Sixteen: Muscle Tension 99
    Chapter Seventeen: Brainwaves 104
    Chapter Eighteen: Medicinal Herbs and Spices 108

Chapter Nineteen: Essential Oils 114
Chapter Twenty: Toxicity 120

Part Three – Mental Considerations 131
Chapter Twenty-One: The Importance Of Belief In The Power Of Belief 132
Chapter Twenty-Two: Mind Programmes And Genetic 136
Chapter Twenty-Three: Acceptance, Forgiveness And Letting Go 150
Chapter Twenty-Four: Stress, Anxiety And Panic Attacks 157
Chapter Twenty-Five: Mindfulness 168
Chapter Twenty-Six: Visualisation And Affirmations 172

Part Four – Emotional and Spiritual Considerations 177
Chapter Twenty-Seven: Negative Emotions ... 178
Chapter Twenty-Eight: Positive Emotions 183
Chapter Twenty-Nine: Spirituality 188

Part Five – In Closing 195
Chapter Thirty: Snippets 196

In Closing 210
…And Finally 212
References 215
Glossary of Terms 218

Introduction

At age fifty-eight I was fit and healthy. A short while later, I wasn't. In fact, I was very ill. I consulted with several NHS doctors over the next few months, all of whom offered me nothing but bewilderment and fear. I then consulted with several allopathic specialists privately, and they all promised to 'get to the bottom of this', but none of them did. Finally, I ventured into the alternative medicine world and did achieve some worthwhile help from two functional medicine doctors, but not enough.

I'll soon be seventy-three years old, and I'm certainly not as fit and well as I was at fifty-eight. From time to time, I've asked myself how different I'd have been now if I hadn't spent close to fifteen years on my recovery journey. Of course I'll never know the answer to that, but I now have a good life, and as I look at people of similar age – and younger–and note how many of them have, arthritis, or diabetes, or heart disease or cancer, or whatever else, and are reliant on complex daily pharmaceutical regimes to 'manage' their symptoms, I feel pretty lucky, and I take no pharmaceuticals.

Three or four years ago I was nothing like as ill as I'd been earlier, but I was far from well. Then, one morning, without knowing why, I thought, 'This is my responsibility, I'm on my own and I have to sort myself out.' And I did. The list below consists of what I believe were the keys to my recovery and could be the keys to recovery from most if not all chronic illness. But to be clear, I'm not talking about quick fixes. What I am talking about is a wide-ranging protocol that I developed via much research followed by months of trial and error that took over a year to bear fruit once in place.

I believe it's very important to understand that it takes a long time to develop a chronic illness, and you don't heal overnight. There are no magic bullets, at least none that I found, but I'm pretty sure that most of those with chronic illness have the potential to heal.

Some of my approach is common knowledge, some is science based, and some is just my opinion, some of which might be considered controversial. Regarding 'my opinion', I won't differentiate by saying 'I believe' or 'I think' at every verse end throughout this book because that would be tedious, but do please bear in mind the 'just my opinion' element as you read.

My list -

1. Your diagnosis is just a label, and being wedded to it can hold you back.

2. Take responsibility. You're in charge. You. Nobody else.

3. There are four elements to you – physical, mental, emotional and spiritual. They must all be nurtured.

4. What you put in, and on your body becomes you – junk in, junk out.

5. Doctors aren't God – what they know is what they've been taught and not all they've been taught is true.

6. Digestion – achieving a well working digestive system is vital. All other physical elements are dependent on that.

7. Water – clean drinking water and lots of it, is extremely important.

8. Supplements. If you take supplements, quality really does matter, so don't skimp on price. If skimping on price is your only option, don't buy supplements.

9. The two key causes of chronic illness are toxicity and deficiency, either physical, mental, emotional or spiritual, or any combination of these.

Yes, it's a short list, totally lacking in detail. There is much need for expansion and clarification, and this book is my attempt to expand and clarify via a series of explanations related to each of the nine items on the list.

So, what will this book do for you? Well reading it will do nothing, but I'm confident that reading then acting on at least some of what you've read backed up by lots of commitment and determination will at worst improve your health and at best completely restore it, regardless of what that illness is.

What this book won't do is refer to or offer suggestions for any particular chronic illness because to do so would be entirely irresponsible. I don't know you, the person reading this book, nor do I know what road you're traveling on or what treatments you're receiving. This book is about beneficial generalities rather than any given illness specific. Yes, these beneficial generalities might be all you need to recover your health, but, equally, they might just provide useful adjuncts to any treatment programme you're willingly engaged in. Either way, I see no downside.

Finally, I must stress that this book is not about acute health issues, that can be efficiently and effectively dealt with by your doctor or a specialist you're referred to. But if you have a chronic illness and would like to get beyond just 'managing' it, feel free to take and put into practice whatever you find useful in this book, but as a responsible adult please be clear that it's for you to take personal responsibility for what you do and what you don't do.

IMPORTANT NOTE – I'm not a doctor and I have NO medical training, and this should be born in mind as you read the pages that follow. I only know what I know from more than fourteen years of personal in-depth research and experience. My expectation is that what worked for me will work for you, at least to some extent. I do not and will not encourage anyone to resist or ignore conventional medical advice if they feel that such advice is the right way forward for them, though aspects of it might well be a helpful adjunct to the advice they're receiving. This book is more for those who aren't happy with the medical system, those who've been through it and achieved little or nothing of benefit, or those who are at least disappointed with what they've achieved thus far. But even if you are such a person, any new symptoms you experience should always be investigated, initially by your GP then, if necessary, by a specialist. Don't assume that such symptoms are related to your existing condition.

Where I refer to a person who could be either sex, rather than constantly saying 'he or she', I've used 'he', not in an attempt to be sexist, but for readability.

Whilst reading, you may come across the mention of something that requires more information. If that's the case, please refer to the references section at the end of the book. Hopefully, you'll find it there.

PART ONE

Preliminary Considerations

Chapter 1 – Desire

Chapter 2 – Kiss frogs

Chapter 3 – Beware of your Label

Chapter 4 – Take responsibility

Chapter 5 – Intuition

Chapter 6 – Glimpses

Chapter 7 – Smile

Chapter 8 – Distraction

Chapter 9 – Doctor knows best…..sometimes.

CHAPTER ONE

Desire

'When a person really desires something, all the universe conspires to help that person to realize his dream' – **Paulo Coelho**

Are you ready to get well, I mean really ready? What a stupid question! Of course you are, right? Well it's just possible that you aren't, as I discovered from personal experience.

The vast majority of chronically ill people want to be well at the conscious level, but for quite a few, there are things going on in their subconscious that are getting in the way. Please understand that I'm not suggesting that these people are 'faking it' or that it's all in their head', because that's not so other than in very rare cases. The reality is that their physical symptoms are as physically real as anyone else's.

So when this is the case, what's going on? There are many ways that your subconscious can scupper you and here are just a couple of examples –

1) There is something going on in your life that you hate, perhaps a job, a relationship, virtually anything, and sickness provides the subconscious with what it needs, a reason to escape that 'something'.

2) You're not getting the attention or love or empathy

that you crave, consciously or subconsciously, and being sick elicits such things from those around you, at least in the short term.

I'd like to emphasise that these two examples along with numerous other possibilities are hardly ever at the conscious level. They're usually the subconscious mind searching for solutions and settling on sickness as an answer.

I'd like to ask you a favour. When you're in bed tonight and just before you go to sleep, will you dwell on this possibility, avoiding denial and being totally honest with yourself as thoughts come to mind? If you'll do that, next morning there's a very good chance that you'll know whether or not this is an issue for you, again as long as you're being absolutely honest with yourself. If you find that it is an issue, don't worry, it can be dealt with.

Okay, you wake up and are one hundred percent sure that you really do want to be well. Great, you're off to a good start.

But now I'd like you to ask yourself a few questions.

1) Is getting well your number one priority?

2) In the short to medium term, are you prepared to be totally selfish, putting all else to one side to achieve your objective?

3) Some of the useful tools to wellness are quite expensive, and money might be short. If you're intuitively drawn to an approach that's currently

unaffordable, are you prepared to review your finances and establish whether there are ways to release the money needed? Are you prepared to give up things that you love but don't actually need, like your smartphone, a pay to view TV network, takeaways or Amazon Prime, for example?

4) Will you make the effort to use comparison sites to save money on utilities and insurance? It really is amazing how much you can save in order to release funds for your wellness campaign.

If your answer to any of 2), 3) and 4) is 'no', then so is your answer to 1).

But if something that you're drawn to really is unaffordable, please don't dwell on it in a negative way. You can still make good progress and you can still get well using the things and techniques that you can afford. It just might take a little longer.

What if you wake up next morning, though, wanting to deny it but deep down knowing that your subconscious is letting you down? Well that's actually good because you've opened a door that needed to be opened. The job then is to consider whatever your issues are and make a firm decision – being sick is a price worth paying or it isn't. I hope you decide that it isn't.

If so, then the need is to face such issues head on and make a choice –

1) remove them from your life. If the issue is your boss at work, for example, change your job.

2) change your attitude towards them. Using the same example, be philosophical about it. Accept that your boss is in charge and that his job is to delegate tasks to others including you. Then carry out those tasks to the best of your ability in a good-natured way. If you can do that, you might be surprised what a positive difference it makes to your relationship. Whatever the issue is, there's always that choice, you can eliminate it or change your attitude towards it. I'm not saying dealing with these things is always easy because it isn't, but with a good, positive approach, it can be done. And when it is, you really will want to be well.

When you've established that you really do want to be well, I'm afraid that you're not quite there. The final step is not to wish or hope that recovery is achievable but to know that it is, and you have to know it is at the very deepest level of your consciousness. There are ways to help if you have difficulties with that, and I aim to consider those in another chapter.

I fully appreciate that for some, total commitment to getting well can be difficult if not impossible, mothers dealing with the requirements of small children, for example. Where this is the case, I have total sympathy, but please don't give up. Get as much help as you can from those around you then work on your health issues with whatever free time you can find. If you do that, positive progress can still be achieved, admittedly more slowly than you'd like, but progress is progress however slow it might seem.

Finally, a good idea is to keep a diary in which you note how things are developing. Then every few weeks, look back at your earlier entries and note the changes in you. Those changes, which you might not notice without your diary for reference, can be truly inspirational because they encourage the desire and determination to continue with the good health creating things that you're doing.

CHAPTER TWO

Kiss Frogs

'Sometimes you have to kiss a lot of frogs before you find your prince.' – **Bianca Frazier**

When I began my wellness journey, although I'd heard of it, I'd never read 'The Princess and The Frog', and I now know that my perception of it, which was that the princess spent her life kissing frogs until one turned into a prince was incorrect. But that doesn't matter.

What does matter is that for reasons I don't really understand – divine inspiration, maybe? – my perception of the story repeatedly came into my mind as I searched for answers. In the early stages of my journey, I knew nothing of healing, and I do mean nothing, All I did know is that I wasn't getting answers from the professionals so I had to find them for myself.

What this means is that my process was entirely one of trial and error – kissing frogs – and the vast majority of the frogs I kissed just croaked and hopped away. But as time passed, I began to find my princes, things that helped me and things that led to other helpful things. My protocol began to develop, and the more frogs I kissed the quicker that development progressed.

Had I not kissed all those frogs, I'd have achieved nothing, and that's why I'm telling you all this. Not all of the things in this book will help you because we don't all need the same things. But if you try them all one at a time then listen to your body, you'll find the ones that do, your princes.

So please don't be put off by the frogs that croak and hop away. If they do put you off, you won't progress. Your princes do exist, and you will find them as long as you persist with determination and count then dwell on your successes rather than your inevitable failures.

So please kiss frogs–and keep kissing frogs until you find the ones you need, whether they be in this book or elsewhere.

CHAPTER THREE

Beware Of Your Label

'To limit your potential, accept the label you're given'–**anon**

I'm sure that anyone reading this book will know what a placebo is, but perhaps not so many will be aware of the nocebo effect. Unlike a placebo, where a substance that has no health benefit improves symptoms because the recipient believes it will, a nocebo can create havoc in your body, mind and emotions on receipt of bad news and/or existing false belief.

For example, you visit your doctor with a set of symptoms, he examines you, notes your symptoms and diagnoses you as having XYZ chronic disease, a disease that you're aware of and what its implications might be. He softens the blow by explaining that although there is no cure, your symptoms can be managed with pharmaceuticals or some other medical protocol. The reason he suggests there's no cure is that he doesn't know the key underlying cause of your 'disease', and you cannot correct something if you don't know what it is – so you get a label that everyone else with your or similar symptoms gets. I must at this point make it clear that your doctor should always be your first port of call and that his diagnosis will most probably be a correct one. What I'm suggesting is not that he's wrong, but that the label you're given can have a strong negative effect on your psyche if you take it to heart, potentially adversely affecting your inbuilt healing ability.

As you leave the surgery, you're understandably upset, you may develop a headache, your legs might feel weak, or whatever, but the point is that you feel worse than you did ten minutes earlier despite the fact that nothing in you has changed since then, other than being given a label, which is the reason you feel worse. That's the nocebo effect, and it's a very strong effect that really can hold you back if you become wedded to it. So, what to do now?

To my mind, if you're chronically ill, assuming you weren't born with damaged genes, or if some part of you is genuinely damaged beyond repair, both of which possibilities are really quite rare, you're either toxic in some way, deficient in something, or somewhere in your body, your mind or your emotions there's an imbalance, usually created by a toxin or a deficiency.

Again to my mind, toxins can usually be eliminated or neutralised and deficiencies can be corrected as can imbalances. If these things can be done, then homeostasis can be achieved, and if homeostasis can be achieved then so can good health and wellbeing. If you understand and accept this, then you don't need the label, and if you discard it then the nocebo will get bored and move out of your life. You'll then be open to the real possibility that your doctor's 'no cure' comment might be flawed.

But hang on, I have my diagnosis, it's what my doctor

says is wrong with me and all my family and friends know that's what's wrong with me. I can't just say I haven't got it anymore.

You're right, you can't when talking to doctors, friends and family, but you can when talking privately to yourself. And if your 'self-talk' is positive and optimistic, it creates belief, and the power of belief, which we'll talk about in a later chapter, is truly amazing. Remember, your diagnosis is simply a label given to a particular set of symptoms – it's a nocebo, that tells you nothing about what's going on in your body or what can be done about it beyond symptom relief.

So, if I accept all this, I'll become well? If you read and act on what you read in this book or perhaps elsewhere, yes that's possible. But sometimes, even often, you do need outside help, possibly from a functional medicine doctor or a naturopath, both of whom seek causes that can be corrected rather than symptoms to be managed, and corrected causes can lead to good unmedicated health.

The purpose of this book is to provide information and ideas that I believe will act as a starting point to your healing journey, a journey that is likely to be more difficult if you believe your label and what your label implies.

CHAPTER FOUR

Take Responsibility

I believe we are who we chose to be. No one is going to come and save you, you've got to save yourself
– **Barry Manilow**

Once you've been given your diagnosis, you can continue with your doctor, or you can see a medical specialist or other practitioner privately. But what happens then? If you're lucky, you'll experience empathy, kindness and understanding, and those things are good because they invoke hope, reassurance and a feeling that help is at hand.

These doctors and practitioners may listen attentively, take notes and nod sagely. But towards the end of your consultation they may make a suggestion then say something like, 'Let's try that and I'll see you again in a month.' – or two months, or three months, or whenever. Then you get into a cycle that tends to progress slowly, perhaps eventually leading somewhere, but perhaps not. And please be aware that they might well suggest something that you instinctively feel uncomfortable with, and that's a red flag because that lack of comfort is your intuition talking, and a wise man always listens to and respects his intuition.

The above just isn't good enough. You deserve much more attention than that. I'm not blaming the doctor or practitioner, and I'm not saying don't consult him. They have many other patients and there are far too few hours in their day. It's unreasonable to think that they'll spend much time pondering on your particular problems.

You might then turn to a partner, a friend or a family member for help, and they may well be more than willing to give it. But the reality is that they don't really know how to help, and however hard they try, their love and best intentions will never be enough to provide all that you need.

What you do need is 24/7 care and attention, and there's only one person who can give you that. You. And accepting that fact can be incredibly liberating. So, if you are to stand a chance of a full, permanent recovery, you have to take responsibility because, quite simply, nobody else will. And in taking responsibility and being totally in charge of your progress, perhaps listening to advice but deciding alone whether or not to take it, you need to put yourself first. In short, you have to be independent and selfish until you're well, and that's not a suggestion, it's a rule!

CHAPTER FIVE

Intuition

'It is always with excitement that I wake up in the morning wondering what my intuition will toss up to me, like gifts from the sea. I work with it and rely on it. It's my partner.' –Jonas Salk

In common with some other ancient religions, for many hundreds of years, Taoism has maintained that we have two brains, one in the skull and one in the gut, each independent of the other and each containing separate and independent compartments. Until relatively recently, modern science has consistently dismissed this belief.

However, in January 1996, it was reported in the medical section of the New York Times, that Western scientists had discovered a network of neurons, neurotransmitters and proteins acting as a single entity of complex circuitry that transmits messages between neurons, enabling it to learn, remember and affect emotions.

This entity was found in the tissue of the oesophagus, stomach, small intestine and colon. It's now official, having been named the 'Enteric Nervous System', and it operates independently of the 'head brain'. For greater clarity, perhaps it should have been called the 'Gut Brain'.

Back to Taoism. So it appears that they were right all along. They believe that the gut or belly brain controls emotions as well as digestion, and that when neurotransmitters go awry, both emotions and digestions are adversely affected, leading to all manner of physical problems. For this reason, they suggest a simple process that, given practice and time, can help bring the neurotransmitters back into balance, thus easing gut and emotional problems, and in doing so, relieving the associated physical issues.

So it's quite possible that this process could be a useful adjunct to your recovery journey, and it isn't difficult to do.

First, lie on your back on any flat surface, bend your knees and keep your feet flat on the surface.

Next, sense how the surface supports your weight, feeling yourself sinking into it, even if it's unyielding.

Next, ensure your hands are warm, and place them on your belly in the area of the navel. Breathe into your hands, so that your belly gently rises and falls. After each exhale, don't immediately inhale. Instead, wait for the next inhale to come naturally, no effort required. Do this for a couple of minutes.

Next, move your attention from your belly to your hands, then to your arms, then all the way back to your spine, then allow the warmth/energy in the hands to expand into the whole abdomen, whilst observing the gentle in and out flow of your breathing.

Next, 'listen' to your belly. Sense it. Is it tight? Is it

relaxed? Is it anxious? Don't try to alter anything, just listen and sense as your belly gently rises and falls. You should soon feel calm. When that happens continue the practice for as long or as short a period as you're comfortable with.

If nothing else, the expansion and contraction of the diaphragm will give some of your internal organs a much-needed massage.

I don't know whether this will help you or not, but I can say it definitely won't if you just try it a couple of times then forget about it. Damaged systems take time and perseverance on your part to heal. But I reckon it's worth a try. If Taoism was many hundreds of years ahead of modern science in discovering this second brain, my thinking is that perhaps their answer to caring for it is too.

Now to the important point of this chapter. Taoism also believes that the belly brain is all knowing and is where intuition comes from. So next time you get a 'gut feeling', don't mess about, go with it, because, clearly, intuition isn't a figment, it's real, and it's incredibly informative.

CHAPTER SIX

Glimpses

'When you catch a glimpse of your potential, that's when passion is born.' – Zig Ziglar

If aiming towards recovery from chronic illness, state of mind matters, and it's as well to understand that the more you dwell on something positive, the better you feel, and the more you dwell on something negative, the worse you feel. That's the law.

For those experiencing a chronic illness, there are lots of negatives, and there's an almost inevitable tendency to dwell on those negatives. That's perfectly understandable, but in terms of regaining good health, it's not helpful.

When I was at my worst, which was over a period of several years, much of my time was spent dwelling on the pain I was experiencing, the malaise, the numerous symptoms, the inability to do the things I'd previously enjoyed, the being left at home when others left to enjoy a good day out, the fall in earning capacity etc.

But every now and then I'd experience a glimpse of normality, albeit a fleeting one. I might wake in the morning feeling pretty normal, but then I'd get up and all the bad stuff returned within minutes or even seconds. Or perhaps I'd be absorbed in something on

TV, and for a short while I'd feel reasonably well.

These glimpses were initially very rare, but when they did occur, I'd feel good about myself, albeit temporarily, because they represented hope, and the possibility that if I could feel like that now I could feel like it permanently. And what I found was that the good feeling I got stayed with me longer if I applied my mind to it. What's more, the glimpses and accompanying good feelings gradually became more and more frequent.

Over the years I've asked quite a few ill people if they experience these glimpses, and 100% of them said 'yes', sometimes following a little thought. Okay, I can't be sure that they're experienced by every ill person, but even if someone eventually says 'no', I'll suspect they may be wrong, because the early ones are of such fleeting nature that they're easily dismissed, or even consciously unnoticed. I also suspect that if they're persistently dismissed or unnoticed, they might throw in the towel and stop coming. So beware.

It's a given that where unpleasant symptoms exist, dwelling on them is the natural thing to do. But if you can learn to notice your glimpses when they materialise and dwell on them with a smile on your face, they're very likely to become more and more frequent, and that must surely be a good thing, possibly even an important step on your healing journey.

So if you do experience those occasional glimpses of the old you, try to embrace them and to concentrate your mind on them. See yourself experiencing more of them, more often and longer lasting. See them as your future. I honestly believe that the vast majority of chronic illness doesn't have to be forever, and that minimising concentration on your symptoms and general malaise, focusing instead on the glimpses, they might just bring those symptoms to an end that bit sooner.

CHAPTER SEVEN

Smile

'Light up your face with gladness
Hide every trace of sadness
Although a tear may be ever so near
That's the time you must keep on trying
Smile, what's the use of crying?
You'll find that life is still worthwhile
If you just smile'

When John Turner and Geoffrey Parsons wrote those words to Charlie Chaplin's melody, they knew what they were talking about.

We all know that a smile or laughter creates positive emotions that support our wellbeing and lift our spirits, at least temporarily. A good smile transforms physiological and emotional chemistry to bring us new energy.

That's all very well, but when you've had a chronic illness for months or years, there seems little to smile about, and it's understandably easy to become a grouch, which leads to spontaneous smiles becoming an absent feature of your life, as do the benefit that a smile brings.

But there is much evidence that a forced smile can alter our emotional state for the better in the same way that a spontaneous smile does. Here's some of that evidence–

In his book, 'The Expression of Emotion In Man And Animals', Charles Darwin observed that, 'The free (forced rather than spontaneous – my brackets) expression of an emotion by outward signs serves to intensify an emotion.'

Also in the 19th century, psychologist, William James, pointed out that emotions are dependent on a bodily state or expression. Change that bodily state or expression and the emotions will change with it.'

Much more recently, researchers Paul Ekman and Richard Davidson found a voluntary (forced) smile actually alters regional brain activity in much the same way that a spontaneous smile does.

In a discussion of their findings in the publication 'Psychological Science', they conclude – 'While emotions are generally experienced as happening to the individual, our results indicate it to be possible for an individual to choose some of the physiological changes that occur during a spontaneous emotion simply by making a facial expression.'

Whilst accepting that unwanted emotions are a part of chronic illness, it seems to me that if those emotions can be improved, even by a little and for a short while, that must be beneficial.

So, I tried smiling whether I felt like it or not, and initially I did feel a slight improvement in mood. But by persisting to the extent that my wife, Hazel, began asking, 'what on earth are you grinning at?', those improvements became more than slight and lasted longer than a short while. I take that as evidence that the people quoted above were on to something.

Every little helps when trying to piece together the chronic illness jigsaw puzzle, and I'm not suggesting that smiling will cure you or eliminate all of your symptoms. But it might help you to try persistent forced smiling whether you feel like it or not. You might be pleasantly surprised by the result. It seems to me that anything with the potential to improve your life in any way at all is worth consideration, and what's to lose by giving forced smiling a try?

CHAPTER EIGHT

Distraction

'The idea is to improve somebody's day. That's how I've always viewed my job. I'm a distraction therapist. I make people's problems go away for just a little bit'–Steve-O

Let's say that you're having a bad day so you're lying on the couch. Your four-year-old daughter is playing in her room upstairs. Suddenly, you hear a series of crashes. You leap from the couch and into the hall where you find your daughter lying still at the bottom of the stairs. Quickly, you phone emergency services. The ambulance arrives as your daughter begins to stir then cry.

Following an initial examination, she's taken to A&E as a precaution, and you accompany her in the ambulance. An hour or so later, other than a few minor bruises, your daughter is declared okay, and the symptoms that had led to you lying on the couch start to return. But for over an hour and a half you hadn't given them a thought. You'd felt alright, your only concern being for your daughter.

Okay, that's an extreme situation that no doubt involved a good slug of adrenalin, but it's also an illustration of the power of distraction.

A less dramatic scenario might be a surprise phone call

from an old friend who you've not heard from for a very long time, and who knows nothing about your chronic illness.

The conversation lasts an hour or so, and by chance, neither of you ask how the other is. Instead, you talk of old times, memories of mutual friends you lost touch with, the week in Spain you shared and the alcohol that got you legless. In short, old and great memories were revisited, resulting in many anecdotes and a great deal of laughter. As you put the phone down, your symptoms, which had been totally absent during the conversation, return, and you realise that for around an hour, you'd felt so much better. That's diversion at work.

The problem is, though, that such diversions don't come along all that often, so neither does the easing of symptoms that they bring with them.

However, if you can find something to do that you really enjoy, and that absorbs you completely, the same reduction of symptoms is likely to occur simply because your mind has been distracted from your illness. With something as unpleasant as chronic illness, it's not surprising that you constantly dwell on it. It's natural and there's no shame in it, but it's not constructive because the more you dwell on unpleasant things, the worse they become.

To create distraction, maybe a hobby that requires your full attention for a while each day is a good way to go. It's certainly worth thinking about the possibilities. Is there something you did in the past that you loved and could go back to? Do you have friends who are keenly interested in something you could join them in? Might something that caught your eye in a magazine be worth investigating? Might you be completely absorbed in that?

Trust me, the ideas are out there, and I'm convinced they're worth investigating until you find the one that's right for you, the one that will distract you from your illness enough to take your mind off it for a while. Doing that can only be beneficial and could be another part of the puzzle, albeit it a small one, that helps you along the recovery road.

Of course, I do appreciate that you may be too incapacitated at the moment to seriously think about hobbies or whatever, because I was in that position for a very long time.

If that is the case, here's what I did for distraction. I came across a website called One Radio Network, that has well over a thousand recorded interviews on many subjects but mainly health issues. These can be listened to online, or downloaded to your computer, tablet or phone, all free of charge.

I spent many, many months listening to these interviews, and they were mostly interesting enough to provide the required distraction. Also, there are a huge number of free podcasts on line, covering just about any subject you can think of. So, when seeking distraction, there's always a worthwhile option, regardless of your incapacity.

In my experience, the more you can turn your mind

away from your symptoms, the less important those symptoms become. Distraction is admittedly a small step, but the road to wellness is really all about 'steps', and sometimes, the smallest ones provide progress that you'd never think they were capable of.

CHAPTER NINE

Doctor Knows Best... Sometimes

The doctor of the future will give no medicine but will interest his patients in the care of the human frame, in diet and in the cause and prevention of disease' – **Thomas Edison**

'The art of medicine consists of amusing the patient while nature cures the disease.' –**Voltaire**

I love that second quote because I'd suggest that in many, many cases it's as true today as it was when it was written over two centuries ago. But the question I'm asking here is, 'Is what your doctor tells you always right?' My answer is 'Maybe, but that very much depends on what he's treating.'

Before I go on, I'd like to stress that I'm confident that the vast majority of students enter medical school with a huge desire to help their future patients, and I'm equally confident that they maintain that desire when they leave medical school to become doctors. But I see two problems which are -

- Medical schools receive funding from pharmaceutical companies, but there's a price to pay for that funding.

- When it comes to specific chronic illness treatment training, the emphasis is almost entirely on the use of pharmaceuticals and surgery, ignoring the many other safe and effective alternative options. I must stress though, that in some areas such as trauma, intensive care and diagnosis for example, the training is excellent as are the results of that treatment.

So, what's the problem with the relationship between medical schools and pharmaceutical companies?

'It is no longer possible to believe much of the clinical research that is published, or to rely on the judgement of trusted physicians or authoritative medical guidelines. I take no pleasure in this conclusion, which I reached slowly and reluctantly over my two decades as an editor of the New England Journal of Medicine.' **– Dr Marcia Angell, a physician and long-time editor-in-chief of the New England Medical Journal (NEMJ)**

'The case against science is straightforward: Much of the scientific literature, perhaps half, may simply be untrue. Afflicted by studies with small sample sizes, tiny effects, invalid exploratory analyses, and flagrant conflicts of interest, together with an obsession for pursuing fashionable trends of dubious importance, science has taken a turn towards darkness' **– Dr Richard Horton, the current editor-in-chief (at the time of writing this) of the Lancet – considered to be one of the most well respected peer-reviewed medical journals in the world.**

So, what went wrong?

At the beginning of the twentieth century there were several successful medical modalities working happily alongside the new medicine of pharmaceuticals. Then two very wealthy people, Messrs Rothschild and Carnegie recognised the potential to increase their wealth even more by expanding the newly created pharmaceutical industry. To do this, they planned to -

- Discredit all the other modalities.
- Invest heavily into expanding the pharmaceutical industry.
- Support medical schools with millions of dollars, but only those schools that specifically taught the use of pharmaceuticals and surgery. No others would be supported with grants or donations.

Within forty years, their plans came largely to fruition and the allopathic system – usually referred to as conventional medicine these days–was firmly at the top of the tree by a very long way. This system is what I think of as the 'medical machine'.

So, what's wrong with the 'medical machine'?

First and foremost, it has little interest in finding cures for chronic illness, which is why I don't support cancer or heart disease charities that are supported, advised by and manipulated by 'the machine'. Rather, their interest is in 'managing' chronic disease, and they're very interested in that.

Why would that be? Curative single or short-term dose drugs would show little profit, whereas drugs designed for management can create a lifetime customer (the patient) providing an unbelievably high profit line – the pharmaceutical industry is one of the most profitable industries in the world, and the vast majority of research goes into developing such management pharmaceuticals.

It's important to say, though, that I'm not suggesting that all medical research conclusions are worrisome. That would be unsupportable because some is valuable in helping people with symptom control, trauma and intensive care etc. But equally, a fair percentage of its conclusions are worrisome, involving fraud in a small but significant percentage of cases, and researcher's preconceived ideas, poor practice or general bias, often due to considerations around current and future funding.

Even if a research group is entirely self-funded, they might begin with a hypothesis they desire to see proven, and that desire may influence their thinking around methodology and other research aspects. I've sometimes read a research paper then compared its content with the summary that reaches the media and have been bemused by the difference between what they actually say.

An example of the type of 'bad science' that doctors so often rely on is the saturated fat hypothesis. This is a case of pure fraud that has perpetuated for many decades. In the 1950s, Ansel Keys believed that saturated fat blocked arteries and, therefore, was the cause of heart disease, and he set out to prove what he believed.

The Seven Countries Study was the result, and it did appear to prove his hypothesis. But he actually studied twenty-two countries, the evidence from fifteen of which did not agree with him. To deal with this inconvenience, he excluded those fifteen countries from the study.

When Ansel Keys presented his study, several other researchers contradicted him, saying that their research indicated that increased sugar intake was the real culprit. Eventually, they were proven to be correct. Now, many doctors still warn us off saturated fat due to its highly exaggerated health risks, seemingly confusing real, clean animal saturated fats with the genuinely harmful trans/hydrogenated fats found in 'healthy' spreads and processed foods.

Also, pharmaceutical research can do cunning tricks with statistics that can make a particular pharmaceutical look more effective than it really is. For example, suppose you have a test related to, say, heart attack risk, and your doctor recommends a pharmaceutical that will reduce that risk by fifty percent. Put like that it surely makes sense to accept the recommendation despite the potential side effects of that particular pharmaceutical, some of which might be quite worrying.

But what if the trial related to that pharmaceutical went as follows –

It was set up properly and ran for ten years. There were

one hundred participants taking the pharmaceutical and one hundred participants taking a placebo. At the end of ten years, two people in the pharmaceutical group have died of a heart attack and three of the control group have died of a heart attack, one more than in the pharmaceutical group. So, that's a fifty percent improvement in the pharmaceutical group, right?

But let's turn things around. Ninety-eight participants in the pharmaceutical group survived and in the placebo group, ninety-seven participants survived, a difference of one in a hundred. Bearing in mind potential side effects, would you have accepted your doctor's recommendation based on that small difference, one that I would consider too small to be scientifically significant?

So, please keep in mind that if reading research papers, it's best to ignore the summary and read the whole thing, which sometimes has no bearing on what the summary says, and most importantly, look into who's funding the research.

Also, throughout allopathic medicine's history there have been numerous cases of accepted wisdom later proven to be wrong, and in some cases, dangerous. Thalidomide springs immediately to mind. Many, many pharmaceuticals have been given the all clear by the relevant authorities only to be withdrawn months or a few years later because of the damage, including fatalities, caused to patients. Many if not most doctors will happily prescribe new drugs based on the glowing reference given by a medical rep whose sole objective is to sell his product. Who knows how many of these new pharmaceuticals will be found ineffective or dangerous at some future date?

In terms of general advice, be wary. For example, we're told we must get our cholesterol and blood pressure levels down to unnecessarily low levels via the use of pharmaceuticals that are known to carry potentially harmful side effects. But do we really need to get blood pressure readings down to 120/80 or lower? And are total cholesterol readings really meaningful? I don't think so.

And low-fat dietary advice to avoid heart disease is still widely accepted. But up until the nineteen fifties, fat was a key food source, and this fat was saturated animal fat. But since the general population switched to plastic artificial hydrogenated and trans-fat spreads, heart disease has escalated at quite an alarming rate.

May I ask you a question? Do you know of anyone with a chronic illness who has been cured by their doctor or a specialist referred to by their doctor? I don't. And by 'cured' I mean back to their old self with no reliance on medications.

Two more points before I close this chapter –

- According to research in the USA, treatment by the allopathic medical system is estimated to be the third cause of premature death, third only to heart disease and cancer. Worldwide, pharmaceutical companies have been fined billions of dollars for various misdemeanours. They pay these fines without complaint because they represent a relatively

- insignificant percentage of their profits.

- Something else that you might not be aware of is that in the USA and the UK, pharmaceutical companies are given immunity from prosecution for the damage their vaccines cause. Instead, both countries have tax payer funded compensation schemes for vaccine damaged people that have paid out millions. We're told vaccines are totally safe, so why do these compensation schemes exist?

Those involved in all of the above have a great deal to do with the training of your doctor, which is why I say, 'Doctor knows best.... sometimes.'

In summary, in some areas of allopathic medicine, trauma related for example, the 'medical machine' can be justifiably applauded, but when it comes to chronic illness, I feel it to be seriously lacking. But I must make it clear that I have respect for most doctors, who are doing the best job they can with the toolbox limitations they're provided with. A lot of good has come from medical science but so has a lot of bad. Not everything your doctor tells you has validity because not all of what those who educate and support him have validity. Do please show your doctor respect, and listen keenly to what he has to say, but keep in mind that he's not God and his advice shouldn't be considered gospel without question. When in conversation with your doctor, I'd suggest using the question 'Why?' to each answer he gives you.

PART TWO

Physical considerations

Chapter 10 – Digestion

Chapter 11 – Diet

Chapter 12 – Water – what you drink matters

Chapter 13 – Two simple ways to super nutrition

Chapter 14 – What I have for breakfast and why

Chapter 15 – Supplements

Chapter 16 – Muscle tension

Chapter 17 – Brainwaves

Chapter 18 – Medicinal herbs and spices

Chapter 19 – Essential oils

Chapter 20 – Toxicity

CHAPTER TEN

Digestion

'All disease begins in the gut.' – **Hippocrates**

For a variety of reasons, many people affected with a chronic illness experience digestive problems. But if you can eat pretty much what you like with no discomfort, and if you have at least one bowel movement a day that leaves your body quickly and easily without discomfort, and is a good colour, light to medium brown, and is well formed, sausage shaped and around twelve to eighteen inches long, feel free to skip this chapter. This is for those who would love to be in your position.

In this book's introduction I said that all the other systems of the body are dependent on the digestive system, and I believe that with a vengeance. And the reason is quite simple.

All of the body's systems rely on the numerous essential nutrients supplied by a good diet and a well-functioning digestive system to maintain themselves and remain healthy. A poor diet and/or a poorly functioning digestive system fail to supply those nutrients, leaving the door open for all manner of sickness and disease. I believe that Hippocrates was right all those centuries ago when he stated what I quoted above, but today, millions of us pay scant regard to that simple truth.

It's often said that you are what you eat, and in the long-lost days of traditional farming and healthy digestive systems, that was probably true. But now we have factory farming, poor quality food, c-section births and formula fed babies, both of which interfere with development of a new-born's essential microbiome. So perhaps now, the saying should be 'you are what you absorb' rather than what you eat, and many, many of us don't absorb well.

The digestive system is incredibly complex, and I should start by saying that I'm not an expert on its technicalities and intricacies because I've never had to put much effort or research into solving the relatively mild digestive issues that I experienced, which were reflux/GERD/heartburn, increased intestinal permeability (leaky gut), and small intestinal overgrowth (SIBO). I must stress that I'm very aware that there will be readers of this book who suffer far more than I did digestive wise, because I know that my digestive issues were quite modest compared to those of many.

With that in mind, my concern is that what I say here may seem patronising, and indeed may be patronising, to those who suffer far more than I did, and especially to those with the more serious and complex problems such Crohns disease, ulcerative colitis, gastric ulcers and coeliac disease etc. This chapter will offer them less value than I'd like. I'd suggest that if you're in that category, you consider consulting with a good functional medicine practitioner, a naturopath, an ayurvedic doctor or even a clinical herbalist who specialises in the digestive system.

For the less serious problems, though, specifically the ones I mentioned above in relation to my own experience, I think it's possible that what I did might help those with more serious versions of these things, because a principle is a principle, and I suspect that the underlying cause of such issues is likely to be the same or similar whether the symptoms are mild, moderate or severe. So, what follows is what helped me but may or not help you.

First, I'd like to cover a few basics that I believe have the potential to at least reduce your symptoms, and quite possibly resolve some of the less serious digestive complaints completely.

1. Very often, almost any digestive issue will respond well to supplemental probiotics and a digestive enzyme complex simply because healthy gut bacteria and a good supply of digestive enzymes are essential to the digestive system, and so many people are severely lacking in one or the other or both for a variety of reasons, a major one being prolonged use of antibiotics.

There are lots of options out there, but two probiotics that I rate highly are Body Biotics SBO bacterial cultures and Bio-Kult. I alternate these to increase the variety of beneficial bacteria strains. A digestive enzyme formula I like is Higher Nature Supergest vegetarian enzymes. I buy all three of these from Bodykind.com. But there is a wide choice of good quality options out there, though I'd suggest being wary of the cheaper offerings.

Fermented foods and drinks can also help.

2. For at least three weeks, apart from grass fed butter, which doesn't tend to cause digestive problems, try cutting out all grains and dairy foods from your diet. Why? because these are major potential causes of gut distress and other complaints that result from such distress, and I've known people who've completely resolved their symptoms by doing this alone. If after three weeks you've seen no improvements, then you can add them back into your diet if you want to.

There are, of course, several other foods that some people develop intolerances to, so if excluding grains and dairy doesn't help, it may well be worth looking further afield. I've heard it said several times that the food you crave most is often the cause of your ills, so although you certainly won't want to, maybe it's worth starting there.

3. Many gut issues are due to low stomach acid. If you drink within around thirty minutes before a meal or around one and a half to two hours after a meal, there is the potential to dilute your stomach acid before it can do its job, so it's worth aiming to avoid drinks within those time scales.

4. Chew your food to pulp before swallowing. Why? First, I've heard rules like chew thirty times or sixty times, or whatever. Well that might be right for some, but not necessarily for you. Whether it's twenty, thirty or sixty times or whatever, the objective is to have nothing solid left in your mouth when you swallow, so the number of chews required is the number that

achieves that. Your gut has a major, energy sapping job to do as it liquidises, extracts nutrients and excretes waste. If it's clearly struggling, chewing to pulp takes some of the strain by providing a good start to the digestive process, and will help it tremendously. One important point, though, is to keep your mouth closed while chewing. If you don't, you'll likely draw in air to your digestive tract, which may slow digestion and possibly cause bloating and wind.

5. Try to leave around twelve hours after your last food of the day and the following breakfast. You like to rest at night and so does your digestive system, so it makes sense to have twelve hours 'on' (gut working hard) and twelve hours 'off' (gut more relaxed). An important caveat is that if you have poor blood sugar control, long periods without food can lead to hypoglycaemia, which is not something you want. So under those circumstances, a twelve-hour break may be too long, in which case just go for as long as you can without feeling weak or ill.

6. Many people say that a weekly fast of eighteen to twenty-four hours will give your gut a really good rest, and that it will love you for it. I've never done that, but I do know of people who have found it beneficial. But again, perhaps not if you have blood sugar control issues.

7. Instead of three meals a day, try five smaller ones. This means that instead of facing three mammoth tasks a day, your gut will face five smaller, more easily and quickly digested ones, and it'll be happier that way.

8. Back to stomach acid–slow digestion can be caused by food remaining in the stomach for too long because gastric juices are in short supply. One way to increase this supply is to try Swedish bitters, which are available from Amazon and elsewhere. If you put a small amount of these bitters on your tongue around ten to twenty minutes before you start eating a large or largish meal, a message is sent to your stomach, warning that there's a big job on the way. The stomach then decides that it had better get to work straight away so it's ready when the meal actually arrives. In fact, anything that's really bitter will help, but Swedish bitters are convenient and designed specifically for this job, and you only need the very small amount of around a quarter to half a teaspoon to put your stomach into 'bring it on!' mode.

9. I know it's not easy, but try the best you can to reduce stress levels – stress alone can cause all sorts of digestion problems because you're autonomic nervous system is in sympathetic 'fight or flight' mode, and when that's the case, blood is diverted away from your gut and immune system (which reduces function) to your muscles. A simple approach that can be quite effective in some people if done consistently, is to find a quiet place twice a day and do ten minutes of slow, deep diaphragmatic breathing. This can switch your autonomic nervous system back to parasympathetic (relaxed) or neutral from sympathetic (uptight). Mindfulness practice can be very effective, too.

10. When you get the urge to go to the loo, act on it as soon as humanly possible, regardless of inconvenience or embarrassment. Stool that stays in the colon for

longer than it should starts to harden, and this can result in chronic constipation. Incidentally, although magnesium oxide is not a good option for the normal benefits of magnesium – see the supplements chapter – it can be very useful if you suffer from constipation and, to my mind, it's far safer than most commercially available laxatives. Start with 500mg a day and work up to a maximum of 2000mg a day. But this option may not be suitable if you have kidney disease. Check with your doctor if that's the case. Once things are moving, I'd strongly suggest increasing your dietary fibre intake by eating more fruit and vegetables and decreasing animal derived foods.

So that's about it. The above are a few basics that I believe are worth experimenting with and which might help, possibly in a big way.

Now to what helped me with acid reflux, leaky gut and SIBO.

Acid reflux

First, some clarification. I see all over the place that acid reflux, Gastroesophageal reflux disease (GERD) and heartburn are treated as being interchangeable names for the same thing, and that's not quite correct. The difference is that GERD is classified as a disease, acid reflux is a mild form of GERD but not considered serious enough to be in the disease category, and heartburn is simply a word to describe the almost inevitable symptom of acid reflux and GERD. I believe that what troubled me for a while would best be described as acid reflux.

The standard medical treatment is to prescribe proton pump inhibitors (PPIs), which reduce stomach acid production. But these are problematic in at least two ways.

First, reflux can certainly be caused by over production of stomach acid, but it can also be caused by too little stomach acid and, possibly, by gas produced by an overgrowth of bacteria in the small intestine. How can that be?

There is a sphincter, a sort of hinged door, that separates the stomach from the oesophagus, and this opens and closes depending on stomach acid levels. When levels rise, the sphincter receives a message to close, thus preventing said acid entering the oesophagus, potentially causing damage. But if stomach acid is too low, the sphincter doesn't receive that message and therefore remains open. So what acid is in the stomach, however little, can easily enter the oesophagus, creating reflux. It is also, I believe, possible that excess gas from too much small intestine bacteria, may force open the sphincter regardless of stomach acid levels.

Secondly, PPIs have been linked to serious adverse effects including Clostridium difficile infection, increased risk of bone fractures, increased mortality in older patients, acute interstitial nephritis, hypomagnesaemia, Vitamin B12 deficiency, rebound acid hypersecretion syndrome, mineral deficiency, community acquired pneumonia, and hyponatraemia, none of which, I'd suggest, you want. For these reasons, authorities now suggest that PPIs should only be used in acute cases and for short periods, but there are many, many people in the UK who have been on them for years.

If you've been prescribed PPIs and have been taking them for more than a month or so, I'd suggest that you see your GP to discuss current guidelines, which he may not be aware of.

Having a healthy level of stomach acid – not too much, not too little – really is important because unless it is, good digestion isn't going to happen. There are three tests that I'm aware of, which are the baking soda test, the betaine HCL challenge test and the Heidelberg stomach acid test. Details are beyond the scope of this book, but you'll find such details courtesy of Mr Google. I will say, though, that the baking soda test is only indicative and the HCL test is more indicative, but not one hundred percent accurate. The plus side is that both can be done by yourself at home and involve minimal cost. The Heidelberg test is the gold standard, but is quite expensive and only available from a private doctor, naturopath or functional medicine practitioner.

So, what helped me apart from the above-mentioned Swedish bitters that I used for quite a long time?

First and most importantly, avoid alcohol, carbonated, sugary and energy drinks, artificial sweeteners, fried foods, spicy foods, vegetable oils other than extra virgin olive oil, and, as much as possible, processed foods.

Second, consider the use of probiotics and digestive enzymes as mentioned earlier in this chapter.

Third, try camomile and ginger teas, both of which

may calm the stomach.

Fourth, don't drink around meal times – see earlier in this chapter.

And fifth, organic apple cider vinegar. This was the biggie for me, but quality is extremely important. If it's nice and clear, it's not good. It should be a little cloudy and have what's called 'the mother' in the bottom of the bottle; shake the bottle and its presence will be obvious. I took a dessert spoon mixed with a little water, slightly sweetened with raw honey about twenty minutes before each meal. I understand that ACV has made matters worse for a very small percentage of people, so it might be a good idea to start with a teaspoon, slowly building up to the tablespoon.

Note – if you're experiencing an acute reflux episode, it's worth trying a quarter to half a teaspoon of aluminium free baking soda in a small glass of water. Bob's Red Mill is a good, clean one, but there are others.

Intestinal permeability (leaky gut)

Leaky gut is where undigested proteins (gluten, for example), toxins and microbes are able to pass through the intestinal wall into the bloodstream, creating all manner of chaos. So to my mind, the need is to tighten up or seal the intestinal walls to the extent that only nutrients can get through.

Strong indications that leaky gut is present are severe bloating, food intolerances, fatigue, joint pain, headaches and general digestive issues. Having these signs doesn't prove that you have a leaky gut, but they are a strong indicator.

First, try the ten suggestions outlined in the above list, and eat a really good diet, paying special attention to avoidance of grains and dairy, because elements of these like gluten and lactose are amongst the very things that can get into the bloodstream when leaky gut is present. Sprouted seeds and fermented vegetables like sauerkraut, for example, can be very helpful, but in both cases, too much initially can be counter-productive, so it's best to start with small quantities and build up gradually.

I was very lucky. I saw slippery elm bark powder recommended on an obscure website, so I tried it at around one tablespoon a day in water, and my leaky gut related symptoms resolved within about a month. I've had no problems since, though I still take it occasionally as a sort of insurance policy. But what's interesting is that I've not seen this recommendation elsewhere, though it certainly worked for me. Perhaps I was just lucky.

However, there are a few commonly used foods and supplements for leaky gut treatment, which are –

High quality Probiotics and digestive enzymes.

High fibre foods like steamed vegetables and fruit, slowly building up to around 40 grams daily.

L-Glutamine, which is well established as a leaky gut repairer.

Marshmallow root powder.

Liquorice root powder – anything up to 6 grams a day, but beware if you have hypertension. If so, use a Deglycyrrhizinated (DGL) liquorice supplement, which shouldn't adversely affect your blood pressure levels.

Collagen, in either powder or capsule form.

I'm afraid leaky gut treatment does involve some trial and error regarding supplements, it being a sort of speculative mix and match approach, but you could always start off with slippery elm bark. Like me, you might be lucky.

Small intestinal bacterial overgrowth (SIBO)

In simplest of terms, this is gut bacteria migrating to areas of the small intestine where they shouldn't be, at least not in high numbers. That doesn't sound too important, but for many reasons beyond the scope of this book, it can create a whole host of problems, perhaps most importantly deficiency in many nutrients including iron, calcium, vitamin B12 and all the fat-soluble vitamins.

I was never tested for SIBO but made an assumption based on the symptoms for leaky gut that are listed above, though there are others too numerous to mention here but available from that nice Mr Google.

I successfully treated it with diet which, to be honest, I didn't follow religiously, and essential oils.

Because traditional effective treatments are in depth and restrictive, perhaps it's as well not to start a treatment programme unless SIBO is confirmed by using what's called 'The Hydrogen Breath Test'. I'm not sure that mainstream doctors offer this, but good naturopathic and functional medicine practitioners do. They would then probably offer a treatment programme of two restrictive diets, one after the other, possibly adding antibiotics or other antibacterial agents, along with supplements to replace nutrient deficiencies caused by the SIBO. But much would depend on what caused the problem in the first place and the severity of symptoms.

This is what I did, based only on personal research –

I ate two tablespoons a day of organic coconut oil for its mild antibacterial capability. I then used the following pure, food grade essential oils – oregano, clove and frankincense. I took them internally, mixed with coconut oil in a capsule, and also massaged over my abdominal area diluted with a carrier oil. I must stress that being 'food grade' is absolutely essential if taking internally. This worked for me, but please understand that mine was a mild self-diagnosed case, so things might be very different in a more serious professionally diagnosed case.

Please note that essential oils can be great healers, but improper use has potential dangers. I'll touch on essential oils elsewhere in this book, suggesting specific further reading.

I must stress that the above suggestions are what helped me, and whether or not they will help you, I really don't know. But I do think that they're worth a try. If they don't help, my advice would be to find and consult with a naturopath or a functional medicine practitioner because in my experience, they're much better at dealing with issues such as these than mainstream medicine is.

Finally, as Hippocrates knew, if you don't sort your digestive system out, you're in trouble whatever else you do. So if you have digestion problems, I'd suggest that dealing with them should be your number one priority.

CHAPTER ELEVEN

Diet

'Let food be thy medicine and medicine be thy food'
– Hippocrates

'The best advice is to avoid foods with health claims on the label, or

better yet avoid foods with labels in the first place.'
– Doctor Mark Hyman

'Life expectancy would grow by leaps and bounds if green vegetables smelled as good as bacon.'
– Doug Larson

Why is a good diet so important? If you are chronically ill, my stance is that you have a toxin or toxins and/or a deficiency or deficiencies. You can have toxic emotions, toxic beliefs, and you can be toxic spiritually, believing that only your religion has validity, for example. Yes, you can be deficient in those areas, too. But here, we're talking about diet. Some people are super detoxifiers and super absorbers, and they are the lucky ones who never or rarely get ill. Their body can handle these things, though as they age, their ability to detox and absorb will inevitably deteriorate.

But most people aren't that lucky, and if you are chronically ill, you are in that group. A good diet is important for everyone, but it's especially important for you, because a good diet increases nutrients, so you reduce deficiency, and has fewer or no toxins for your body to deal with.

So what is a good diet? Below are my seven 'right diet' tips for most people -

1. As much as you can, avoid junk or processed foods, which means anything from a restaurant, but specifically anything from a fast food restaurant, or anything in a box, packet or tin.

2. Eat a 'real food', ideally organic, plant-based diet. 'Real food' meaning as nature intended it to be.

3. Eat your vegetables and salads raw as much as you can without creating digestive discomfort.

4. Don't over-cook plant foods.

5. If you can stomach them, eat fermented foods.

6. Add as much colour to your diet as you can.

7. Other than that found in fruit and vegetables, avoid sugar, and especially sugar substitutes.

Why minimise, ideally eliminate, processed food?

I'll assume I don't have to explain why junk food is a bad idea, but in most cases, processed food, which is the staple for most people in the Western world, isn't much better because it almost invariably contains preservatives, unnatural flavour enhancers, sugar or artificial sweeteners and God knows what else. These are all toxins. They're not toxins that will kill you in the short term, but small amounts of toxic material build up over the years if you're not a good detoxifier, and over time they can do a great deal of harm. In my opinion, they have much to do with the frightening acceleration of chronic illness in the Western world.

I know many people can't face the concept of not eating from a box, packet or tin, and if that's so in your case, please at least look at the ingredient list on the packaging and avoid anything that includes an unfamiliar ingredient. At the very least, research that ingredient. The chances are that you won't like what your research reveals. Please be aware that 'natural flavouring' can mean pretty much anything, and is very often far from natural. So don't be fooled by that or anything else that 'sounds' okay.

Some higher end grocery stores are now selling much cleaner processed foods, but they're still far from ideal, and they tend to be quite expensive, costing quite a lot more than preparing the same meal yourself.

So the vast majority of processed food is toxin rich and nutrient poor, but let's not be too obsessed. Straying into the processed arena now and again isn't going to kill you. It's the daily use of these foods that present the potential long-term dangers. Try to make such straying the exception rather than the rule.

Why a real food plant-based diet, and why organic?

I'm an omnivore, so why do I suggest a plant-based

diet? The clue is in the word 'based'. I don't mean vegetarian, I mean an absolute minimum of fifty percent plant food, and preferably sixty percent plus, or ideally around eighty percent organic vegetables, fruit, nuts, seeds and legumes etc. This is because that's where most of what your body needs comes from.

So why eat any meat at all? Because there are some important nutrients that are hard, sometimes impossible, to find in plant food, such as vitamin B12, the omega three oil DHA, vitamin D3 and the amino acids creatine, and taurine, for example. Yes, vegetarians (and vegans) can supplement with such nutrients, but wherever possible, I think it's best to get them from real food. However, you can certainly overdose on animal foods, and I believe that if they represent around twenty-percent of your diet that's more than sufficient to provide adequate supplies of said nutrients.

But importantly, your animal products should come from pastured animals that eat their natural diet – grass in the case of beef and lamb. Why? First, there is the cruelty issue. Factory farmed animals live in awful conditions. They have a life, but one that's really not worth living. They're also fed with unnatural foods and, of course, those foods become them, which when you eat them, become you, at least in part. Additionally, they're often given antibiotics as a matter of course in order to limit the diseases related to cramped conditions. And finally, they're regularly injected with hormones to promote growth which enables quick turnaround from birth to market. So, truth be told, you really don't know what you're eating when it comes to factory farmed animal foods.

Animals reared and fed in the traditional way, however, may have a relatively short life, but it's a happy life that, if we didn't eat them, they wouldn't have at all. Also, unlike factory farmed animals, they provide us with healthy saturated fat, which our bodies need and which are the ideal choice for cooking.

Pastured, organic animal products are quite expensive, but I feel that the average person eats too many animal products anyway, many of them processed. If that average person dramatically reduces consumption of the processed options and reduces to some extent the non-processed, the savings made can be utilised to purchase adequate supplies of the pastured, organic options.

Incidentally, as well as fat, including butter, from traditionally farmed animals, good quality saturated fat can also come from avocados and coconut oil. For things like salad dressing, though, I'd suggest using high quality extra virgin olive oil.

So why is it important to eat organic plant foods as much as possible?

Because if they're not organic, plant foods will have been sprayed with a host of chemicals–pesticides, fungicides and herbicides. You do not want these things in your body. And sadly, washing doesn't help much because these chemicals get inside the plant as well as on it.

Many 'authorities' state that non-organic food contains equal nutrient value to that of organic. If that's the case, why have many nutrients in most of the food we eat declined so much since factory farms became our main food source? Also, I believe that most organic farmers tend to farm using traditional or close to traditional methods, so they regularly replenish the nutrients in the soil that their crops are planted in. Additionally, some of these nutrients need to be broken down or even created by the healthy bacteria that live in the soil, but the weed killer used in factory farming will kill many if not most of these bacteria.

I believe that organic food is quite widely available in the USA, but I appreciate that a wide variety of organics can be hard to find in some areas of the UK, including where I live. To get over this problem, I use two companies that do nationwide home deliveries, and both of whom carry a huge range and variety of organic food. They are Riverford Organics and Abel & Cole. No doubt there are other such companies that I'm not aware of. I know that supermarkets carry a limited range of organic foods, but I'm a little suspicious of these. They look too perfect and clean, and I wonder what they're washed in. But that might just be me being a bit neurotic.

I do appreciate that for many, eating an organic, or even a partially organic diet isn't financially viable. With that in mind, perhaps it's a good idea to be aware which fruits and vegetables are the most and least heavily sprayed with pesticides, herbicides and fungicides, so that if you wish, you can adjust your diet accordingly.

Various sources state that -

The most heavily sprayed non-organic foods are – strawberries, spinach, nectarines, apples, peaches, pears, cherries, grapes, celery, tomatoes, sweet bell peppers and potatoes.

The least heavily sprayed organic foods are – avocados, sweet corn, pineapples, frozen peas, onions, papayas, eggplants, asparagus, kiwis, cabbage, cauliflower, cantaloupes, broccoli, mushrooms and honeydew melons.

Why eat as much raw plant foods as possible?

If you cook non-animal foods, their Vitamin C is destroyed, essential enzymes are destroyed, any fat content is changed into unhealthy trans fats, sometimes called hydrogenated fat, and in some cases, around fifty percent of any protein is destroyed. Consequently, they're not nearly as nutrient rich as they were when raw, and they may now contain a toxin via the trans-fat. Clearly, some vegetables like broccoli, for example will upset a few stomachs if eaten raw, but others, like carrots, for example, are fine. All salad ingredients are eaten raw, and all fruits can be. So to maintain a high intake of raw food isn't difficult.

I mentioned the loss of enzymes above, and this is an important issue. You are born with a large supply of enzymes that are essential if all your body's systems are to function efficiently. As you age, your supply diminishes and your body doesn't replace them adequately. Replacement enzymes in quantity have to come from food, and that food has to be raw.

Why not over-cook plant foods?

As mentioned above, many people have difficulty digesting some raw foods, but by not over cooking, you can retain a reasonable percentage of their nutrients. It's certainly not a good idea to boil in water because many nutrients are left in the water that you then throw away, and cooking in the oven will leave them pretty much nutrient deficient. Steaming is the way forward, and five or six minutes at full steam is more than adequate to render them digestible for the majority of people.

Why eat fermented foods?

There are numerous fermented foods, the most popular probably being yoghurt because it tastes good. But please don't buy the low fat highly processed ones that come in all manner of flavours, most of which are artificial. They are junk food. Buy full fat Greek style, preferably organic, and if you want to flavour and/or sweeten it, that's fine – use fruit and perhaps a splash of organic maple syrup or raw honey.

Other less pleasant tasting, at least to me, options that are extremely healthful are kefir, kombucha, sauerkraut, pickles, tempeh, natto, kimchi, miso and some cheeses if they haven't been pasteurised – read the label.

Okay, so why are fermented foods so good for you? The fermentation process creates billions of beneficial bacteria, which can populate your colon, adding quantity and variety. These have the potential to improve your digestion in general and nutrient creation in particular because some nutrients are actually created by your gut bacteria. If you eat enough fermented food, there's no need for supplemental probiotics. But as hinted earlier, most fermented foods really don't taste that good, so the temptation is to try them once but never again. And if you eat large amounts before your gut is acclimatised, an upset stomach is quite possible. So if you want to try some of the more exotic options, start slow and build up gradually, allowing your taste buds and digestive system to get used to and appreciate them.

Why add lots of colour?

I'm talking about fruit and vegetables here. Different colours indicate different nutrient combinations, so the more colours you have, the wider variety of nutrients you get. If you look around, you might be surprised just how many different coloured fruits and vegetables there are. There are even purple carrots now, for goodness sake.

Why no sugar or sugar substitutes?

Sugar has zero nutritional value. It makes you fat, and it confuses your pancreas and liver, quite possibly leading to metabolic syndrome then type 2 diabetes and, possibly, heart disease and cancer.

But what's so bad about sugar substitutes? Well let's look at the most commonly used one – Aspartame. This is a non-food chemical compound found in hundreds of processed foods and drinks. It has been linked to the development of several serious health conditions including cancer, diabetes, heart disease and brain disorders. It can't possibly do you any good in any way, and it has the potential to do a great deal of harm over time. That's just one, and I'd strongly advise against using any chemical sweetener because they're all bad in one way or another. Incidentally, be aware that aspartame is sold under several names, so if you use an artificial sweetener, you may well be taking aspartame unknowingly.

Something to keep in mind

If you light a fire, you benefit from the warmth it creates. But you also generate toxic smoke. Fortunately, this goes up the chimney and doesn't hurt you, though its environmental effect is a different matter. When you eat, you obtain nutritional benefits. But you also generate 'toxic smoke' in the form of free radicals from the metabolism of the food you've eaten, and these free radicals are seriously harmful. Fortunately, and assuming you're eating well, your food contains antioxidants that can neutralise your 'toxic smoke'. However, if you eat too much food, you can exhaust your antioxidant supply quite quickly, leaving the free radicals able to cause havoc throughout your body. It's therefore a good idea to eat slowly, note signs of satiation and stop eating when they appear.

Be patient

The benefits of a good diet don't become immediately apparent because when a healing nutrient reaches a cell that needs that nutrient, you're only just starting the healing process. That process can take days, weeks, months or, in rare cases, even years. So please don't give up if you feel no immediate benefit, always keeping in mind that true, natural healing always takes time.

Finally, I should stress that this chapter is just my opinion of what a good, healthy diet looks like, and I understand that it's difficult if not impossible to follow these ideas one hundred percent of the time. So if this approach makes sense to you, I'd suggest following it as closely as you can without beating yourself up when you lapse, because we all have lapses. I certainly do. I guess the key point is that any improvements you make to your diet, even small ones, will be beneficial, possibly improving your health quite dramatically.

Important note

If you have moderate or severe digestive issues and are being treated by a specialist or alternative therapist who has advised a specific diet, then you should continue to follow their advice until your issues have resolved.

A short note on trying to lose weight

A well-established reason for gaining weight or having difficulty losing weight is eating too many carbs such as bread, cakes, pasta, rice etc. I wouldn't argue with that, and I agree that carb reduction makes good sense.

However, I believe that another major reason for weight gain is a poor-quality diet. Why? When the body is getting low on the nutrients it needs, a hunger signal is sent out, so you eat. But if you're eating low nutrient foods, the body may well persist with the hunger signal because the nutrients it craves haven't arrived, so you eat again, and again. What I found, having realised that the benefits of eating high nutrient food far outweigh the pleasure derived from eating a burger or deep fried chicken, was that the more I ate high nutrient foods, the fewer hunger signals I received, and I now eat far less than I did when eating poor quality food, and I rarely feel really hungry.

But having said that, it's important to appreciate that we're not all the same, and occasionally, you come across interesting anomalies. One I came across a couple of years ago was the case of a woman who was very much over-weight and just couldn't lose the excess, despite doing all the right things. In the end it was suggested she try removing each item from her diet, one at a time for three weeks. When she cut out carrots, she immediately started to lose weight at the rate of around a pound a day, and she achieved a healthy weight in about three months. Who would have believed that – carrots for goodness sake. It's a strange world we live in!

CHAPTER TWELVE

Water... What We Drink Matters

'Drinking water is like washing out your insides. The water will cleanse the system, fill you up, decrease your caloric load and improve the function of all your tissues' – **Kevin R. Stone**

Your body composition comprises mainly of fat, muscle, bones and water. To be healthy, the water content should be in the region of fifty-five percent, though this is variable depending on your sex and fat/muscle ratio because muscle holds more water than fat does. So, if you have a high fat to muscle ratio, your water content will be lower. If you're female and a little overweight, forty-five percent plus water is a reasonable target.

There's nothing wrong with a cup of good quality tea or coffee because they both have benefits of their own, though if you add milk, sugar or artificial sweeteners, those benefits are minimised, and coffee should be avoided if you have fatigued adrenal glands. But your main liquid intake should be pure, clean water. Please, please, please avoid commercial sugary drinks and artificially sweetener laden 'diet' drinks, which are the last thing your body needs, and at least while you're recovering, avoid alcohol.

So what should your daily intake of water be? The

commonly used textbook answer is for every two pound of body weight drink one ounce of water, so if you weigh 140lbs, for example, you need 70oz of water. Incidentally, I add a small pinch of fine Himalayan salt to my drinking water to provide a wide range of minerals. The quantities of these minerals are small but worthwhile. If you try this, the water shouldn't taste salty. If it does, reduce the size of your 'pinch'.

As a generalisation, I guess the above calculation is okay, but we don't all have the same body composition and we don't all have the same requirements. I think there are two better ways to assess your needs –

1) Monitor your pee – if it's consistently a light cardboard colour, you're doing okay, but if it's consistently darker and possibly a bit smelly, you need to drink more water. Please note that certain foods and supplements can colour your pee. For example, beetroot can turn it red and some B vitamins can turn it bright yellow, sometimes with a green tinge, but that's nothing to worry about.

2) Use a set of body composition bathroom scales. Prices range from around fifteen pounds to over a hundred pounds. These measure your body's fat, muscle and water percentages, and if you're getting a readout of around fifty-five percent water or forty-five percent plus if you're female, you have nothing to worry about. I suspect that these scales are less than brilliantly accurate, but their accuracy is probably near enough for this purpose. But please don't obsess about the fifty-five/forty-five percent figures. Reasonably close is okay.

Earlier, I said 'pure, clean, water', and that requires some explanation.

Tap water, and in many cases bottled water is neither pure nor clean. UK tap water contains chlorine, and some water authorities also add fluoride, which is not necessary to maintain healthy teeth. Both of these chemicals block receptors of cells that require iodine, and iodine is a mineral required by many of the body's systems, not just the thyroid gland. And fluoride can be extremely toxic if too much is taken at once.

In addition to chlorine and fluoride, tap water may contain heavy metals, some of which are neurotoxins, pesticides and herbicides along with hormones and pharmaceuticals excreted in the urine of other people. Admittedly these are in minute quantities, but minute quantities add up over the years if you're not a good detoxifier. Also, if you're male, a steady intake of female hormones, however minute, really isn't desirable.

There have been numerous tests on bottled waters, and in many cases, they were found lacking, often containing chemicals, numerous pollutants like bacteria, fertilizer and industrial chemicals. Also, plastic bottles can leach chemicals into their contents, especially in warm weather. Then there are the environmental considerations associated with plastic, of course. Anyway, if you're buying the more expensive and trustworthy glass bottled varieties, they work out very expensive over, say, a year.

If you drink tap or bottled water, at best, your body has to clean it up before it can utilise it, and this involves expending a lot of energy and stressing your liver. At worst, you could be slowly damaging every cell in your body.

Of course, if you're fit and healthy, your body can deal with all these things, though even then, there may be long-term unwanted consequences. But if you're chronically ill, removing them as best you can will help your body heal.

So, what can you do about it? Well there are several possibilities ranging in cost and efficacy, some of which follow -

1. Boiling your water for around twenty minutes then cooling before drinking will kill most bacteria and dissipate much of the chlorine, but little if anything else. This method is inconvenient and not very efficacious, but it's cheap and it's better than doing nothing.

2. Adding a pinch of around an eighth of a teaspoon of vitamin C to a glass of water will neutralise much of the chlorine whilst providing a useful antioxidant dose to your diet. Cheap ascorbic acid is fine if it doesn't upset your stomach. If it does, use sodium ascorbate.

3. Jug filters – these do pretty much and perhaps a little more than boiling does and are much more convenient. The jugs are quite cheap to buy, but ongoing, filter replacement is a cost that doesn't apply to boiling, though the filters aren't overly expensive. So, a better option than boiling but a bit more expensive.

4. Whole house filtration systems like reverse osmosis, for example. These will get your water pretty much as clean as it can be, and your bath/shower water will also be clean. But they're very expensive to buy and install. Also, regular filter changes are essential because there have been many reports of bacterial infestation in them, and like the system itself, these filters are expensive. So they're very good but with serious short and long-term cost implications.

5. Water distillers – I had one of these before I bought what I have now. There are plenty of cheap, nasty ones out there, but a good quality one will cost in the region of two hundred pounds. They do need a regular carbon filter change, but these are very cheap to buy. They produce totally pure water. So why did I get rid of mine?

   a) the process is very slow.

   b) cleaning is a faff.

   c) the water is totally pure but it's also dead. I added minerals salts to mine, but these aren't cheap, and getting the quantities right is a pain. Many people highly recommend these but I don't.

6. There are several pretty good counter-top systems available priced from around two hundred pounds, but after a great deal of research, I settled on The Berkey Filter System, and four years on, I'm delighted that I did.

This system removes the vast majority of everything you don't want whilst leaving what you do want in place. Once set up, which takes about fifteen minutes, the only chores are to wash the bottom section out once a month, which only takes a few minutes, and to clean the filters about twice a year, or more often if you're filtering pond water. The two main filters that come with the unit last about ten years assuming average usage.

My water authority adds fluoride, and if yours does, you'll need the extra fluoride filters, one attached to each of the two main filters, and at the time of writing, these cost sixty pounds for the pair and last for around eighteen months. There are several sizes of the main unit available and I chose the Big Berkey, which is suitable for a family of four and costs around two hundred and fifty pounds. That may seem a lot, but if you need the fluoride filters, and assuming an eighteen-month filter life, which I've found to be about right, the total running cost is around seventy-seven pence a week, and I'd call that a bargain for covering the needs of four people. If you don't need the fluoride filters, the annual running cost is zero for around ten years, at which point replacement main filters will cost ninety pounds at current prices, and these will cover you for the next ten years.

Since buying the Big Berkey, I've been delighted to see that three people who I have great respect for, scientist and researcher Chris Masterjohn, scientist and researcher Mike Adams and cancer survivor, researcher and lecturer on natural cancer treatments, Chris Wark, have all recommend Berkey as the best option for providing clean, pure water.

So that's my choice. Your choice is for you to decide of course, but I would urge you to do something to get the best benefit that you can afford from the one thing that you can't live without for more than a few days. Doing something, even the smallest thing has to be better than doing nothing.

One final point – unless you have guts of steel, drinking iced water is a bad idea because it shocks your digestive system and disrupts the digestive process. Water is best drunk at room temperature.

Footnote

It strikes me that I've just done some serious Berkey virtue extolling and that might raise perfectly reasonable suspicions regarding possible commercial interests. So I'd like to make it quite clear that other than as a customer, I have no relationship with either the manufacturer or any of the retailers and that, therefore, I gain no benefit, financial or otherwise, from recommending it.

CHAPTER THIRTEEN

Two Simple Routes To Super Nutrition

'Nutrition is so important. It can't be stressed enough.' – Dwayne Johnson

'Our body is the only one we've been given, so we need to maintain it; we need to give it the best nutrition.' – Trudie Styler

'Popeye was right about spinach: dark green, leafy vegetables are the healthiest food on the planet. As whole foods go, they offer the most nutrition per calorie.' – Michael Greger

When I wrote the diet chapter, I was conscious of the fact that for many with chronic illness, achieving a perfect or near perfect diet regime isn't easy or even practical for several valid reasons, including feeling dreadful while trying to manage a household and having limited funds due to being unable to work. So when that's the case, are there any ways to dramatically increase nutrient intake which, if the cost of a couple of pieces of equipment is affordable, are economical to do? Well there are two that I think are excellent, and they're what I'll talk about here.

Sprouting

A broccoli seed is much smaller than a pinhead, yet given nothing more than water in its early growth phase, it eventually becomes a large broccoli head, and we all know how good broccoli is from a nutrition point of view. So how does it do that? That tiny seed is packed with a huge number and variety of nutrients and enzymes, so much so, that pound for pound, the sprouts produce at least fifty, yes fifty, times more nutrient value than the fully matured broccoli.

How can that be? Well by the time a broccoli seed has matured into a broccoli head, most of its inbuilt nutrients have been exhausted. But when we eat the very young sprouts, most of those nutrients remain. I've used broccoli as an example, but there is a wide variety of seeds available for sprouting, each offering its own high nutritional value.

So, how do you go about sprouting?

There are several sprouting methods, the equipment for some of which is ridiculously expensive. But for one person, you can provide a week's supply with just two jars. You can even use jam jars, but getting the drainage angle right can be a problem, as can getting the right number of drain holes in the jar's lid. For that reason, I suggest a small outlay on a pair of A Vogel biosnacky germinator seed jars, which have a lid with appropriately sized drainage holes and an extending piece for standing the jars at the correct draining angle. These are widely available, and at the time of writing, Amazon have a pair costing less than fifteen pounds. That is the total cost of your equipment.

Seeds can be organic or inorganic, and the difference in price really isn't significant, so I'd go with organic.

There are dozens of seed possibilities, but to keep things simple, I'd suggest starting off with GEO broccoli sprouts and GEO Andante sprouts, which are a combination of mung beans, alfalfa seeds and radish seeds, together providing a good nutritional mix. These can be bought from several places, but I get mine from www.ukjuicers.com. The broccoli seeds might appear quite expensive, but they produce the most nutritional value of all sprouts, and a box lasts for ages.

So how do you go about sprouting with the two-jar approach?

First, keep in mind that the Andante takes around five days to mature, and the broccoli takes around six to eight days.

Day 1 – Add a dessert spoon of broccoli seeds to a jar and half fill it with clean water. Cover with a cloth to keep the light out for around twelve hours. Rinse and drain the seeds then half fill the jar with water and cover again for a further twelve hours. At the twenty-four-hour stage, covering becomes unnecessary, so discard the cloth. Rinse and put the uncovered jar upside down at the angle provided by the lid in a light place but not in direct sunlight.

Day 2 – Still with the broccoli seeds, rinse, drain and stand as before twice a day, the rinses being around twelve hours apart.

Day 3 – As day 2

Day 4 – Start the same process with the Andante seeds

From then on, rinse, drain and stand as before twice a day until maturity. After a couple of days, at each rinse, stir both jars with a fork to prevent clumping. Hulls and seeds that haven't taken will come to the top, run a slow tap into the jars and these waste products will overflow into your kitchen bowl. When the jars are reasonably tightly full of sprouts, remove and put in a sealed container in the fridge, where they'll keep for about five days. Wash the jar well ready for the next round. Using the two-jar system will provide a useful daily supply of super nutrition.

The above may sound a bit complicated, and if it does, please forgive me for making it so. But once you've established a routine, it really is simple, and the whole thing takes less than ten minutes a day. Just one final point – after three or four days, the broccoli sprouts may develop what looks like a white fungus, but it isn't fungus, and will wash away with the rinsing.

Smoothies

When I first started making smoothies, the only blender that did a really good job was a Vitamix that costs from around three hundred to seven hundred pounds depending on the model. These are amazing machines and I still use mine for making oat milk and lemon juice amongst other things.

But times have changed. Nutribullet were first on the scene with a model that works really well, at much lower cost than the Vitamix, but others have followed, Ninja being an example. Having worked with these, I've found that if you prefer a really smooth texture, it's as well to go for a model that has at least a 900W motor and preferable 1200W. But the less powerful ones will still provide the nutrients you're looking for, albeit not quite so smoothly. If I was seeking a reasonably priced smoothie maker today, I'd investigate the ranges of the two manufacturers mentioned above – Nutribullet and Ninja.

The major benefit of smoothies is that all the nutrients are retained but in a very digestible way, meaning that they are easily absorbed by the body, so they're especially good if you have gut issues. Juicing provides similar nutrient value, but I do have concerns regarding the sugar content. Smoothies retain the ingredient fibre content, so the sugar content is absorbed more slowly than that in a juice, and this reduces the potential for blood sugar spikes that can make your pancreas unhappy, possible leading to type 2 diabetes.

Regarding ingredients, I describe my daily smoothie in the breakfast chapter, but would note here that I don't use much fruit. The only reason for that is that I eat lots of fruit, mainly berries, and so use the smoothie for nutrient rich things that I wouldn't otherwise eat.

In general, though, I'd suggest thinking in terms of creating a green base to which fruits can be added, preferably berries, avoiding strawberries unless they're organic, and perhaps apples and carrots, keeping the really sugar rich fruits like pineapple and banana to a minimum. Some people like to add yoghurt, and that's fine.

Many people won't continue with the smoothie habit

if the taste isn't reasonably palatable. And whilst I think it's important to have a green base, most green vegetables aren't very tasty in a smoothie. For that reason, by all means experiment, but I'd start off with either spinach or kale, both of which blend well with any fruit content. Alternatively, there are some good mixed greens powders available these days, and using those keeps things simple.

A good tip is to buy your fresh ingredients when they're on their sell by date and have a price reduction, then freeze them straight away. They'll keep in the freezer for several weeks. Over time, this can save you a lot of money, and it's been established that frozen fruits maintain their nutrient value.

So there we have it, two ways that take little effort to instigate, yet dramatically boost your nutrient and enzyme intake. With the sprouting, once you've established a routine, each rinse takes less than five minutes, and you can make the average smoothie in less than ten minutes, including clean up. Even If you decide to only try one of these suggestions, you'll still get far more easily absorbed nutrients than you would otherwise, and the more nutrients you absorb, the quicker you'll heal.

CHAPTER FOURTEEN

What I Have For Breakfast And Why

'I rely on breakfast to give me a kickstart of energy in the morning, so I choose my foods accordingly.'
– **Mikaela Shiffrin**

'Like love, breakfast is best when made at home
– **Gina Barreca**

I was once reading a book by a well-known American doctor, in which he said there was more nutrient value in a commercial cereal's box than there is in the cereal itself. That amused me at the time, but although there was a tongue in cheek element to his words, there is some truth in them, too. These cereals are mostly nutrient deficient and heavily sweetened with sugar or even artificial sweeteners. Then there are the non-food additives that you've never heard of. So I'll start this chapter by saying that a bowl of commercial cereal is not a healthy breakfast, though I should say that there's no problem with a bowl of traditional porridge as long as it's sweetened, if indeed you want to sweeten it, with something like raw honey or organic maple syrup rather than sugar.

Currently there is quite a bit of controversy regarding breakfast, with quite a few people stating that you should only eat between twelve noon and eight pm. I can't speak for anyone else, and it may make sense for someone else, but if I did that, I'd get very light headed and might even faint. So I'll stick with my preference for a healthy breakfast.

My thinking is along the lines that while I quietly sleep, my body is hard at work digesting what I've eaten during the previous day, detoxing, seeking and eliminating toxins, healing, rebalancing and so much more. All this activity requires the utilisation of many nutrients. Therefore, my assumption is that these nutrients need some serious topping up, and that's what I aim to achieve at breakfast time.

So this is what I do -

Preparation

I have a lock-and-lock container that's about the size of a cereal box. When the previous batch is depleted, I fill the box with roughly equal amounts of the following – pumpkin seeds, sunflower seeds, sultanas, walnuts, brazil nuts, pecans, hazel nuts, almonds and raw coconut flakes. Preparation time is around fifteen minutes, and the full box lasts a little over three weeks, so that averages out at around five minutes a week preparation time.

Weekly, using my trusty Vitamix, though any powerful blender would do, to 900ml of pure water, I add a lemon, a teaspoon of ginger powder, and a quarter teaspoon of ascorbic acid. I process this at full power for about two minutes then pour the result into a one litre glass bottle, which I then keep in the fridge. Preparation time is around five or six minutes and the bottle lasts a week.

Also weekly, and again using the Vitamix, to 400ml of pure water, I add 30 grams of sprouted oats and a good splash of one hundred percent pure, organic maple syrup and blend for around two minutes. This produces a pure and healthy oat milk. The commercial oat milks I've come across are neither pure nor healthy. This goes into a 500ml glass bottle, which I also keep in the fridge. Preparation time is around five or six minutes and the bottle will last a week, but I spread it over six days.

Daily, I make a smoothie with the following ingredients – 300ml of pure water, two teaspoons of golden linseeds, one teaspoon of hulled hemp seeds, two teaspoons of chia seeds, one teaspoon of hemp protein powder, one teaspoon of Ceylon cinnamon powder, half a teaspoon of turmeric powder mixed with black pepper in a roughly 80/20 ratio, one heaped teaspoon of mixed greens powder, an apple and a clementine. For the mixed green powder, I use Amazing Grass, green superfood with sweet berry, which I buy from Bodykind.com, but there are a few other good brands available.

Morning routine

I give the litre bottle containing the lemon, ginger and ascorbic acid infusion a good shake then pour around one seventh of it into a large glass, top up the glass with pure water and drink.

I add two tablespoons of the box contents to a bowl then add a small handful of cranberries and around one sixth of the well shaken bottle of oat milk to soften the bowl's contents, and eat.

Drink the smoothie.

Note – I buy a large quantity of fresh organic cranberries when they're available around Christmas time and freeze them. They last until around June. For the rest of the year I use organic dried cranberries.

The why

Basically, it's about getting a huge boost of nutrients to replace those lost during the night. I believe that minerals and omega oils are more important than vitamins in the morning because I get plenty of vitamins during the day. So that's what I concentrate on, though there are some vitamins involved. What follows is a brief review of these nutrients -

The lemon, ginger and ascorbic acid mix.

Lemons have several health benefits, but have you noticed that your first pee of the day tends to be darker than at other times? If so, that's because your body is busily trying to dispose of the toxins released during the night. For this reason, your body is a little acidic when you wake up. Lemons are alkalising and that's the main reason I make this drink.

Throughout the night, our digestive system has been busy digesting yesterday's food. The ginger gives your digestive system a little boost to help with the job of digesting breakfast.

I add the ascorbic acid simply as a safe and effective preservative, though it also gives you a small of vitamin C.

The bowl contents.

Pumpkin seeds contain worthwhile amounts of manganese, vitamins B and K, zinc, phosphorous, magnesium, potassium, copper and iron.

Sunflower seeds contain worthwhile amounts of vitamins E, B1, B3 and B6, manganese, copper, magnesium, selenium, folate, zinc, iron and potassium.

Sultanas, contain worthwhile amounts of calcium, potassium, magnesium, vitamins B6 and K, and iron, though I really use these to provide a little sweetness.

Walnuts contain worthwhile amounts of protein, fibre, omega three fatty acids, magnesium, potassium, phosphorous, vitamins B1 and B6, folate, zinc, iron, manganese, and copper.

Brazil nuts contain worthwhile amounts of protein, fibre, selenium, phosphorous, copper, magnesium, manganese, vitamins E and B1, zinc, calcium, iron and potassium.

Pecans contain worthwhile amounts of healthy monounsaturated fats, protein, fibre, vitamins E and B1, manganese and copper. And they're my favourite for taste!

Hazel nuts contain worthwhile amounts of magnesium,

potassium, phosphorous, vitamins E, B1, B6, folate, and K, zinc and copper.

Almonds contain worthwhile amounts of protein, fibre, vitamins E, B2 and B3 magnesium, potassium, manganese, calcium, copper and zinc.

Raw coconut flakes do provide a good amount of fibre and a little zinc, but I add them to provide a little bit of healthy sweetness.

Cranberries are high in antioxidants, they're great for the urinary tract, they support the immune system, they're anti-inflammatory and have anti-cancer properties.

I use sprouted oats for the oat milk simply because sprouted grains are far more easily digested than unsprouted grains. The maple syrup is purely for sweetness, but it does contain a few minerals, and relative to other sweeteners, it has a low Glycaemic index score. I think it's perfectly healthy if used in moderation.

So overall, we have a good supply of protein and fibre, a very good supply of the important minerals, and a reasonable supply of some of the important vitamins, in a really healthy and easily digestible form.

The smoothie ingredients.

Golden linseed, AKA flaxseed, contains omega 3 fatty acids, protein, fibre and a host of minerals, albeit in quite small quantities.

Hulled hemp seeds contain omega 3, 6 and 9 fatty acids,

protein, fibre, vitamin E, manganese, magnesium, phosphorus, zinc and iron.

Chia seeds contain high amounts of fibre, protein and omega 3 fatty acid as well as various minerals and healthy fats. They're famous for boosting energy.

Hemp protein powder contains magnesium, calcium and potassium, but I use it for its high levels of plant protein.

Ceylon Cinnamon powder is full of antioxidants and is anti-inflammatory. Please note the word Ceylon. Other types like Cassia can be toxic if used regularly.

The turmeric powder/black pepper combo is anti-blood clotting, anti-inflammatory, is good for joint pain, and has anti-cancer properties.

The mixed greens powder contains wheat grass, barley grass, alfalfa, spinach, spirulina, chlorella, broccoli, various berry extracts and so much more, providing a really powerful nutrient and antioxidant mix.

The apple and clementine contain fibre and a variety of nutrients. To my mind, apples are a true superfood.

I take a close to one hundred percent organic approach to what I eat, though I appreciate that it isn't practicable for everyone to do that. But even a totally non-organic approach can still provide lots of nutrients and is still very worthwhile. However, if you include a non-organic apple in your breakfast mix, I strongly advise you to peel it, because non-organic apples are very heavily sprayed with pesticides.

So, am I suggesting that you must eat the same breakfast that I eat to regain your health? Absolutely not. I've outlined my breakfast in detail purely as an example of a nutrient dense breakfast option. What I am suggesting, though, is that when you're planning your breakfast, consider the quality and variety of nutrients it will provide, bearing in mind the extra need for those nutrients first thing in the morning, then perhaps make manageable adjustments in order to maximise your intake of those nutrients as much as you can.

Now I have a confession to make. If you're an attention to detail person, you might have noticed that the oat milk was said to last a week, but that I suggested using a sixth of it each day. Well I'm afraid there's a reason for that. Every Thursday, I go to the local Premier Inn and have a full English breakfast. Why on earth am I, this diet fanatic, telling you that? I'm telling you that because I truly believe that even when aiming for a really clean diet, there's nothing wrong with the occasional treat, and I love a full English breakfast. In order to clear my conscience, though, I do have my breakfast smoothie later in the day.

So although I'd love you to be eating a really clean heathy diet because I know your health will benefit if you do, if you slip off the wagon now and then, to my mind, that's okay. It's often said that a bit of what you fancy does you good, and I'm not going to argue with that.

Now, in case you're interested, I'll briefly touch on what I eat and drink for the rest of my cheat free days.

For sipping throughout the day, I have a one litre glass drinking bottle by my side. This is full of pure, water to which I add one or two drops of lemon essential oil, and a pinch of Himalayan salt. The lemon essential oil is for alkalising and the salt is to provide a few extra minerals.

At around mid-morning, I have a nice mug of strong black coffee. But I'd advise against this if you have adrenal fatigue issues.

For lunch, seven days a week, I have a giant salad, including on my full English breakfast Thursdays, but then, I have it later in the day instead of my normal late afternoon meal. The salad consists of a large bed of mixed salad leaves to which I add cucumber, tomatoes, sweet mixed peppers, beetroot and sprouted seeds. With this, I have cottage and Feta cheese. Additionally, I may add half an organic cheese and vegetable pasty or half an organic homity pie, and occasionally, I might add melted cheddar cheese on wholemeal toast, both organic or, and here's my second confession, a mini pork pie. To drink, I'll have green or matcha tea.

In the late afternoon, I have a cooked home-made meal, which will be either a curry, a beef stew or chilli, with loads of green vegetables, either broccoli, cabbage, cauliflower or runner beans, or a combination. I follow this with berries, usually blueberries and blackberries but occasionally raspberries, or cherries, with a big dollop of full fat Greek yoghurt. To drink, I'll have camomile tea. About once a week, I'll switch to organic poached eggs on organic wholemeal toast as a treat.

For snacks, I use un-sulphured apricots (brown, not orange), dates or nuts.

Finally, I regularly remind myself that, from a health point of view, what I eat defines what I become, and I think that such reminders are a good thing.

CHAPTER FIFTEEN

Supplements

'If a potato can produce vitamin C, why can't we? Within the animal kingdom only humans and guinea pigs are unable to synthesize vitamin C in their own bodies. Why us and guinea pigs? No point asking. Nobody knows.' – **Bill Bryson,**

Many doctors and others will tell you that all supplements do is provide you with expensive urine, and that you get all the nutrients you need from diet. If I'd been writing this book fifty or sixty years ago, I'd probably have agreed with them. But today, I think they're wrong.

Since then, intense farming techniques, diminishing soil quality, modern processing methods and delays in getting food to market from far and wide, have created food that is far less nutrient dense than in the past. So I think that for most people, supplements can be of value, in fact great value in many cases, but there are a couple of problems -

The key thing I learned during years of researching supplements, is that quality is everything. My best guess is that around ninety percent of the supplements currently available in supermarkets, pharmacies and health food stores are of poor quality, containing synthetic ingredients that your body doesn't recognise as food. Also, a great many of them are manufactured in the Far East in factories that you'd be concerned about if you saw them. This doesn't apply to all the Far Eastern manufacturing plants, but it does to many, and it's hard to establish which are okay and which aren't. The high-quality options are more expensive, sometimes substantially so, but to my mind, it makes sense to buy one that's efficacious rather than two that don't work or don't work very well. As I said in this book's introduction, if good quality isn't available to you due to financial restrictions, it's better to do the best you can with diet.

Problem two is that there are hundreds of different supplements on the market and it would be irresponsible to detail most of them because I don't know you, the reader, or your condition or which medications, if any, you take. Many supplements are unsuitable for those with certain conditions and equally many can interact adversely with medications. This means that if I recommend a supplement that I personally like, it's possible that it could harm you in some way.

So here, I'll mention just a few that I use on a daily basis and that I believe would benefit the vast majority of people and are extremely unlikely to harm anyone. If you'd like to study the whole subject of supplements, there a several books available on Amazon or from any good book store.

Below is my list of eight safe and efficacious for all supplements in some detail -

Methylsulfonylmethane (MSM)

MSM is a major metabolite of DMSO, and DMSO has been used for decades, orally, topically and intravenously to tackle hard to deal with chronic illnesses, like lupus, diabetic ulcerations, scleroderma and all types of arthritis, for example. It has been heavily researched and found to have many healing properties. It's an analgesic, an anti-inflammatory, it dilates blood vessels, it eases many types of pain and muscle spasms, it easily passes through cell membranes and the blood brain barrier, meaning that it's available to the whole body, it's anti-parasitic and it can normalise the immune system, for example. The list of potential benefits goes on and on, but it's not perfect. Used for any length of time, the user can develop a rotten fish odour, and some users have developed liver and/or kidney problems. It can be bought on Amazon, but I'd never use it without the support of a professional who is expert in its use and the potential damage it can cause.

MSM however, has many of DMSO's benefits without the potential downsides, other than one minor one that I'll come to later. Unfortunately, there has been little scientific research into MSM, probably because it's not patentable, but there's a huge amount of anecdotal evidence from users regarding all manner of benefits, though there have also been some 'this stuff's useless' comments, but I think I know why.

In the late 1990's I bought a book called 'The Miracle of MSM', which seemed well researched and informative. So much so, that I bought some MSM capsules, which I much later found to be a mistake. After around three months of taking the capsules, I'd felt no benefit at all, so I stopped taking them and forgot all about MSM.

It would be between four and five years ago that I heard an interview with a guy called Patrick McGean who, with his wife, had been running what he calls 'The Sulphur Study' for around fifteen years. This isn't a scientific study, it simply receives anecdotal reports back from two hundred thousand (that was then, there may well be more now) participants using a particular type of MSM. The list of positive reports received is endless but includes – chronic constipation resolved, more vivid dreams, morning erections (in the men!), memory returning to dementia patients, people leaving care homes and returning to their own homes, men with erectile dysfunction no longer needing Viagra, older women no longer needing vaginal lubricants, years of chronic pain resolved, and arthritis patients no longer needing medication. These are just a few of the reported benefits. There is no way to scientifically validate anecdotal reports, of course, but they do exist in their thousands.

Mr McGean explained that the reason for these results was that MSM transports much needed oxygen through all the body's cell membranes directly into the cells. This creates energy and allows the cells to excrete their toxins, which the sulphur in the MSM then sulphates and escorts from the body in the normal way. In effect, the MSM is a master detoxifier of the whole body including the brain, but, and this is very important, the oxygen it carries isn't from the air you breathe, but from the water you drink, so you must drink lots of water –

see the calculation in the water chapter of this book. The amount suggested there is an absolute minimum if you want to achieve the best results from MSM.

Earlier, I mentioned one minor downside, which is that some people can get quite a nasty detox reaction when taking MSM. The reason for this appears to be that they're taking enough to get oxygen into the cells and release toxins, but not enough to sulphate the toxins out, so they remain in the blood stream causing the reaction. The answer to this isn't to stop taking the MSM, but to increase the amount being taken.

He went on to say that MSM in capsule form is ineffective, which reminded me of my previous experience. The apparent reason for this is that the capsules contain several excipients, including silicon dioxide, which blocks the sulphur uptake. He also pointed out that most powder or crystal MSM is polluted, and in many cases very harsh chemicals are used in the manufacturing process. These are MSM from a chemical makeup point of view, but they're largely ineffective from an efficacious point of view.

I was quite impressed by all this, and so was, Patrick Timpone, the interviewer. So much so that he agreed to take the MSM for two weeks at the standard dose, which is two heaped teaspoons a day taken approximately twelve hours part, then invite Patrick McGean back for a second interview. During that second interview, Mr Timpone discussed the benefits that he'd found. This specific form of MSM is now for sale on the interviewer's website, and has attracted hundreds of positive reviews, which you can see on One Radio

Network.

I'd have bought some at that time, but including carriage from the States along with potential import duties, the cost was prohibitive. But then one of my favourite UK health product websites, Ancient Purity, started to stock it, and I've been using it ever since.

So what benefits have I found? The first things I noticed were stronger nails and hair, and that I began to recover my libido. Then I realised that the last of what the doctor's called my fibromyalgia disappeared, as did the arthritic pain in my left knee and left forefinger. I was sleeping deeper, though not longer. And finally, the energy I'd forgotten I'd ever had returned to a measurable extent. Please don't think this happened overnight, but most of it happened within six months, and some became noticeable within two to four weeks.

It isn't cheap, and for that reason I've tried several other makes, but they were all ineffective apart from one. That one is KALA health OptiMSM. I don't rate it as highly as the Ancient Purity offering, but it's pretty good and it's half the price, so it is an option.

Finally, if you decide to try this, there are two further things to know – 1) It is quite bitter, but you soon get used to that. 2) If, say, after three weeks, you've felt nothing, first, are you drinking enough water? If you are, increase the MSM dose. It's totally non-toxic so you can take as much as you like.

A multi vitamin/mineral supplement

These will provide a small amount of many of the

things your body needs on a daily basis. I think of them as an insurance policy.

There are dozens of makes on the market, but the vast majority have synthetic ingredients and contain fillers and anticaking agents etc that your body doesn't want to deal with. They are, in my opinion, pretty useless. But two that I like very much are Ancient Purity multi vitamin and mineral complex, available from Ancient Purity, and Terra Nova living multi nutrient complex, which I get from Evolution Organics. Both are food state for maximum absorbency and both are free of binders, fillers and other excipients. The Ancient Purity one would be my first choice based on quality, but that's very much reflected in the price. The Terra Nova is almost half the price, and is fairly close to Ancient Purity in terms of quality. Both are a worthwhile addition to a good diet, each with a very wide variety of nutrients derived from real food, but please don't think that they replace a good diet. They don't. Nothing does. That's why they're called supplements.

Vitamin C

Vitamin C is a great antioxidant that gives back oxygen molecules to other antioxidants that have been stolen by free radicals, thus giving these other antioxidants a new lease of life. It also helps with heart health and immune system function, amongst other things.

As with multi-vitamin/mineral supplements, there are dozens of types and makes available, mostly containing ingredients you don't want.

Nobel prize winning Dr Linus Pauling, who lived into his nineties, spent decades researching and documenting the numerous benefits of vitamin C, and throughout these decades he used vitamin C in the form of ascorbic acid. I decided that if it was good enough for him, it was good enough for me, so generally, that's what I use.

It's available everywhere but I've found that Ancient Purity supply the best and purest version. It's in powder form, which mixes easily in water, and it's completely free of unwanted additives. I take three grams a day. However, it is a little harsh for those with sensitive stomachs, and if that's so in your case, I'd suggest sodium ascorbate as an alternative, again in pure powder form. A worthwhile tip in establishing your needs is to increase your dose daily until you get loose stools, then reduce daily until your stool is back to normal then stay on that dose.

So ascorbic acid is my choice for daily use, but if I have an infection of some sort, or if there are a lot of infections around, I also take liposomal C. This is around five times more efficacious than ordinary C, because whilst ordinary C is water soluble and can't get to everywhere in your body, liposomal is fat soluble and can. The problem, though, is that the commercial offerings are ludicrously expensive. But there is a solution.

There are many videos on You Tube showing how to make your own liposomal C, most of them insisting that you need a jewellery cleaning machine to mix the ingredients and this is a tedious process. I don't agree that that's necessary. If you have a powerful blender you can make your own quickly and easily by mixing 300ml of water with 35gms of sunflower lecithin and 25gms of ascorbic acid for one minute three times with a twenty- minute gap between each time to avoid overheating. This lasts well in the refrigerator so can be available for when needed. I must stress though that the blender does need to be a powerful one. I use a Vitamix S30. You can try this with a less powerful blender, but if the ingredients separate in storage, then I'm afraid the blender isn't powerful enough.

I do accept that the commercial liposomal C is probably a little more efficacious than what you can make at home, but doing it yourself costs a tiny fraction of the commercial varieties and the end result is still very powerful.

Fish oil

Due to the DHA and EPA omega 3 fatty acids it contains, fish oil has numerous health benefits. It's good for your heart, your brain, your eyes, your immune system, your skin and hair and so much more, but there are problems.

First, if you buy it as a liquid, it does not taste good, and that's likely to put you off. For that reason, I prefer capsules. Second, due to general pollution, so many of the products on the market are 'dirty'. Third, although a bottle might say 1000mg of oil, that's not what matters. What does matter is the concentration of the omega 3 oils. Very often, the EPA and DHA content is minimal.

So, when looking for a good option, there are two key

issues to consider – purity and omega 3 content. After much research, I settled on Maximum Omega 1300mg from the supplement company Nature's Best. This has gone through a five-stage purification process and each capsule contains an amazing 715mg of EPA and an equally amazing 286mg of DHA. If shopping around, look for similar levels to that and always check for purity.

Vitamin D (as D3)

Every cell in your body has receptors for vitamin D, and if that doesn't tell you that your body needs it, I don't know what does.

If you can expose yourself to the sun for around twenty minutes a day, wearing very few clothes and no sunscreen oil, you'll get all the vitamin D you need, as long as your body has sufficient cholesterol, which is needed for absorption of D. But very few people can do that, which explains why so many people are vitamin D deficient, especially those living in the northern hemisphere. Some can be obtained from certain foods like oily fish and eggs, but not enough, and that's why I believe that most people should supplement. Incidentally, vitamin D isn't really a vitamin, it's a hormone.

There are two types of supplement available, D2 and D3, and I'd recommend D3 simply because it's much more bioavailable than D2. I take 4000iu a day, though in the past I took much more in order get my levels to where I wanted them. There are lots of good quality D3 supplements around, but I especially like that from the

American company Doctor's Best.

If you'd like to get your levels tested before supplementing, which is a good idea, there's a simple pin prick test that your doctor can provide. However, he's likely to be happy if your blood levels are around 50 nmol/L, whereas I'd be much happier at 80 to 100 nmol/L.

A final point on D3 – D3 is fat soluble, which means it stays in your body for a long time. The cost difference between, say, a 4000iu capsule and a 2000iu capsule is minimal. So if, for example, you want to take 2000iu a day, buy the 4000iu option and take one every two days. You'll save a lot of money over time. And, of course, if you only want to take 1000iu a day, take 4000iu every four days. The point is, buy the highest iu value you can find, divide by the dose you want, and the answer you get tells you how often to take it.

Vit K2 mk7

If taking D3, it's a very good idea to also take K2 in the mk7 form. Why? D3 increases the absorption of calcium, and if you have too much calcium in your blood there is a danger of arterial calcification, and you don't want that. But, equally, you don't want to decrease your calcium intake from food, so you need to ensure that your calcium goes to your bones rather than to your arteries, and that's what K2 mk7 does. It escorts calcium to where it belongs. Clever, eh? I like NutriZing K2 600mcg one a day, available on Amazon.

Magnesium

Magnesium is a mineral essential for most of your body's systems. For example, magnesium is important for energy production, for calming the nerves, for helping digestion of food, relaxing nerves, improving sleep and so much more. But most people are deficient, in some cases dramatically deficient.

If your diet is really good, you may be getting all the magnesium you need, but for most people, I feel that supplementation is a good idea, and it can't do any harm; if you take too much for your body's needs, you'll simply get loose stools. I'd avoid tablets and capsules because they invariably contain things that you don't want, so my recommendation is pure powder, which mixes easily into water or a smoothie.

Avoid the cheapest options like magnesium oxide (unless your objective is to treat constipation, in which case this is the one to use), chloride and carbonate because they provide little or no benefit and can cause digestive problems including diarrhoea in some people. There are a few options like chelate, threonate and orotate that are extremely well absorbed by the body and are of very high quality. But they're also quite expensive and probably not really necessary for most people. As a cheaper but very worthwhile option, I mix a 50/50 combination of magnesium citrate and magnesium glycinate, taking roughly a half a teaspoon a day, and that's what I'd suggest to combine efficacy and affordability. If that creates loose stools, reduce your dose a little each day until your stool is back to normal. I like the NOW brand, which is available on

Amazon.

Transdermal application is a good idea, too, and for that, the cheaper magnesium versions are okay because they're not having to bypass the digestive system. There are plenty of good quality spray bottles on the market and they're not overly expensive. You can also make your own by mixing one-part magnesium flakes into one part of pure, clean boiling water. When dissolved, cool and pour into a spray bottle. Transdermal application can be very useful if you have muscle aches or pains in a particular part of your body.

Please note – if you have kidney disease, check with your doctor before supplementing with magnesium.

Hawaiian Spirulina by Nutrex.

Why spirulina in general and Hawaiian by Nutrex in particular? Spirulina is a true superfood that has far too many health benefits to go into here, so suffice to say that it nourishes the body throughout. The problem is, though, that there are issues with almost all of the products on the market in terms of quality and production methods. Yes, the organic ones are free of pesticides and herbicides, but that doesn't make them pure. They can have a high bacteria count, heavy metal pollution, be heavily processed and can be polluted with animal fertilizers.

The Nutrex Hawaiian offering is grown on the Hawaiian island of Kona in fresh aquifer water then chill dried ensuring maximum levels of vitamins, minerals, antioxidants and phytonutrients. It is transferred from farm to bottle under rigorous quality control procedures, and is totally pure for maximum benefit.

The dose for maximum benefit is three 1000mg tablets a day, and in my experience, the best UK supplier for price and service is a company called Bodykind, who offer a discount scheme based on points per purchase, a price guarantee and extra discounts if you buy two or more bottles at a time. Delivery is free in the UK on orders over fifteen pounds.

So that's my 'safe eight', but I must make it clear that I'm not suggesting that you must take all of them to resolve your health issues. Neither am I saying that if you take these you'll need nothing else. So much depends on your circumstances and particular health problem. What I am suggesting is that the above provide many valuable health benefits individually or in concert, and are unlikely to cause harm regardless of your health status or medication intake.

To investigate the use of supplements further, I'd strongly suggest a consultation with a well qualifies naturopath or functional medicine doctor.

Finally, I'm not specifically endorsing the product providers mentioned in this chapter, it's simply that having tried numerous companies over the years, I've found that these provide very high-quality supplements backed by exceptionally good service. You may find others that are equally good.

CHAPTER SIXTEEN

Muscle Tension

"A tense mind creates tense muscles, and tense muscles hurt!" – **anon**

Do you look like a gormless ape? Fear not, I'm not attempting to insult you. Gormless apes tend to have loose jaws with mouths slightly open, creating an impression of gormlessness. Their arms hang loosely at their side and swing as they roam around seeking out whatever it is that gormless apes eat. Their joints are healthy and flexible, free from the restraints of tight muscles. Basically, their bodies are calm and relaxed. So if you look like a gormless ape, congratulate yourself, you don't have the issue this chapter discusses.

In my experience, most people who are chronically ill tend to be chronically stressed whether they realise it or not, and their chronic stress almost invariably leads to chronic muscle tension, again, whether they realise it or not. And this can lead to aching or painful muscles, low energy, joint pain because the relevant muscles aren't supporting the joint properly, headaches, eye strain and more.

A simple way of establishing if this applies to you, is where you're now standing or sitting, ask yourself, are your shoulders raised, however slightly? Are your top and bottom teeth touching, can you sense tension in your jaw? Do you have discomfort in your temples? Are your fists clenched, even slightly? Are you aching anywhere in your body? If the answer to any of these questions is 'yes', then you're a typical chronically ill person and I think it makes sense to work on this problem, a problem that's delaying your healing journey.

Muscle problems aren't always down to stress, though. They can be the result of mineral deficiency, specifically magnesium and potassium. I'm happy to supplement with magnesium – see the supplement chapter – but less happy to supplement with potassium, as too much can be a bad thing, occasionally resulting in kidney damage. So I prefer the dietary approach to potassium. The chances are that a good diet will provide your needs without risking overload. Lots of foods contain potassium, but a few of the common ones are bananas, potatoes, dried apricots, peas, avocadoes, spinach, wild caught salmon and beetroot. Also, there are specific muscle diseases like muscular dystrophy, for example, but these are relatively rare, and not dealt with here.

So there are three possibilities that warrant consideration, but as mentioned earlier, the most likely is tension induced by stress, which is what we're considering here. Fortunately, there are things you can do about that, which with practice can make a big difference, not just to your muscles, but to your whole body. So let's look at those things now.

First, I have found from personal experience that where an individual has become a chronic muscle tenser, it can take some time and concentration to find resolution.

There's no quick fix that I know of that doesn't involve relaxant drugs, which to my mind aren't ideal for most people because they just provide symptom relief, and they may have unpleasant side effects for some.

But that time and concentration can pay dividends and are, therefore, worth the effort. The basic objective is to, over time, teach yourself to recognise and quickly release any muscle tension that isn't part of a necessary physical activity.

The commonly recognised way to relax the body's muscles is to tightly tension each muscle group then 'let go', feeling the tension evaporate. The idea here is that in releasing the tension you've purposefully created you'll also release the tension that was already there. I have no doubt that for healthy people, this can be effective, but it's an approach requiring quite a lot of energy production, and those with a chronic illness tend to have limited spare energy. So I'm not inclined to suggest this approach despite the fact that it's recommended everywhere. But if low energy isn't an issue in your case, you may well find it helpful.

For most chronically ill people, I've found that vigilance and regular gentle practice bring best long-term results, though I'm afraid that such vigilance and gentle practice may need to continue for a while before relaxed muscles become your subconscious norm.

By vigilance, I mean that, initially, what I'd describe as stage one, the need is to be almost constantly scanning your body for tension when you're up and about. Are your shoulders raised? Are your teeth touching? Is your brow creased? Are you failing to mimic a gormless ape?

In doing this, it's very helpful to enlist the help of those close to you. Ask them to keep an eye on your brow and your shoulders, which should be sloped, not parallel to the floor, and your arms, which should be hanging loose rather than flared out, even slightly. Obviously, if you're standing, your leg muscles will be necessarily tensed, and if you're lifting, then so will your forearms, biceps and back, so you have to be a bit sensible. But continuously ask yourself, is this muscle tense because it needs to be, or simply because I'm tensing it? Eventually, with regular attention you'll soon learn to recognise unnecessary tension and then quickly release it.

For stage two, I'd recommend regular twenty to forty minutes sessions of lying down comfortably so that no muscles need to be tense. Spend a few moments clearing your mind of thoughts as best you can, and getting into a comfortable abdominal breathing pattern, with your stomach gently rising and falling, aiming for a breath rate of no more than one breath every five seconds. Then, starting from the crown of your head working towards your feet or vice versa, it doesn't matter which, monitor what's going on in your body. If starting with your head, are your eyebrows closer to each other than they need be? If so, gently widen the gap, releasing tension in your forehead. If starting with your feet, gently wiggle your toes then let go. Are your feet splayed outwards (relaxed), or are you holding them erect (tense)? If tense, let the tension go so that your feet naturally splay outwards. Continue like this throughout the whole body–lower legs, thighs, buttocks, lower back, upper back, shoulders, abdominal area, hands, arms, face and neck etc. Are your arms lying loosely by your side with your fingers slightly curled? They should be. Is your head 'loose'? If you stood up, would it flop to one side? It should.

I won't go through every muscle group in your body, but, hopefully, the above illustrates the concept.

At the end of the session, when each muscle group is relaxed, any pre-session pain or discomfort should have eased, if only a little, and that's a good measure of your success.

Also, at the end of said session, lie still for a few minutes, learning to recognise what relaxed muscles feel like so that, in future, you'll know what you're aiming for. But don't anticipate perfect relaxation on your first or early sessions. If tense muscles have been your norm over a long period, re-educating them will take time. But they can be re-educated, and when they have been, the benefits will be clear. Eventually, you'll look like a gormless ape, and that will be cause to be proud of yourself.

Finally, if you have difficulty with this routine, perhaps due to wandering attention or boredom, or whatever, recorded sessions led by someone with a calm voice may suit you better. I can highly recommend 'The Body Scan CD set' from Breathworks.

CHAPTER SEVENTEEN

Brainwaves

'The primary goal of Brain Wave Vibration is to help you return to a simple state of being, a place where you can experience yourself and the world without thought or judgement.' – **Ilchi Lee**

What are brainwaves?

When the brain's neurons connect with each other, many thousands at a time, they communicate via small electrical currents that travel throughout the brain's circuits. This creates electrical pulses that in turn create measurable waves. I'm not a neuro-scientist and that's a simplification, but if you want a more detailed explanation, you'll find one via Mr Google.

So why does that matter?

At any one time there will be a combination of these waves depending on what you're doing, physically, mentally and emotionally. But again at any one time, a particular brain wave may be overly dominant, disrupting a healthy balance. If that's so, emotional and neuro-physical health problems may develop.

So what, specifically, are these brain waves?

There are five known wave patterns, four of which have been thoroughly researched and one that is still under investigation but attracting much interest. These are -

Beta waves (13 to 40 Hertz) This is the awake and alert state, the state you want to be in when there are tasks to do, when there are problems to solve, when you need to be alert, when there's an important decision to be made and when you need to be really focused.

Alpha waves (6 to 12 Hertz) This is the relaxed state when your brain is effectively resting, perhaps when you're engaged in a hobby or are engrossed in a good novel. Basically, when you're calm with no immediate worries and when all is good in your world.

Theta waves (3 to 7 Hertz) Perhaps you've been watching TV and it's nearly time for bed. You're starting to lose concentration on the programme and your mind is starting to drift. That's Theta starting to become dominant. It's a state where intuition can come into play and where strange thoughts or images might come to mind, pleasant or unpleasant. Theta tends to stay with you as you slip into sleep, but then begins to fade, though it can come to the fore again during dreams or just before waking.

Delta waves (0.5 to 3 Hertz) This is the deep sleep wave, the dreamless phase when you're totally at rest and totally unaware of your surroundings. This is the wave during which your body heals and rejuvenates. It can also become dominant during a deep, expertly achieved meditative state.

Gamma waves (40+ Hertz) This is the one that, at the time of writing still seems subject to continuing research. Until relatively recently it was dismissed as 'spare brain noise'. But there is a growing consensus that being in a Gamma state improves cognition and mental focus. It's also believed by some that it may positively affect perception and consciousness, may be a natural antidepressant and might even help with ADD and ADHD.

Note – the Hertz ranges above vary slightly depending on who you're asking.

Okay, but what's the benefit of knowing all this?

Imagine it being time for bed, but your mind is busy mulling over the day's events or worrying about tomorrow, or whatever. Or perhaps you need to be alert because there are important issues to be dealt with, but all you want to do is sleep. These are just examples of your brainwaves being out of balance and dominated by a particular wave that's unsuitable for your current purpose. I suffered from this sort of imbalance, and I know that many others do, too. But the good news is that there are ways to bring things back into balance, helping you to sleep well when the time is right or, conversely, be focused and alert when you need to be.

What are those ways?

Some years ago, I bought a piece of kit called the Photosonix Inner Pulse. This has numerous options for guiding your brain into the wave pattern you want, and it does this by creating sound in the form of binaural beats and combining that sound with a light cycle, creating the brainwave pattern that you want. The kit is comprised of a control box, a pair of stereo headphones and dark glasses that emit the light.

This was a transformational Godsend at the time, producing great results, and I still use it from time to time to this day. The build quality is excellent. Sadly, my model no longer exists. But there are lots of other makes and models: just Google 'mind machines.' I do feel that such machines are the quickest and most effective option for adjusting your brainwaves, but there is a problem of price. They range from around two hundred pounds upwards.

Fortunately, there are much cheaper options to achieve the same thing. I have a CD set called 'Brainwave Symphony' by Jeffery Thompson, and this works quite well when used with stereo headphones. It consists of four CDs, one for each of the main brainwave patterns.

Also, if you Google 'brainwave altering downloads', you'll find lots of possibilities. I have no experience of these, but have no reason to suspect that they're not effective, as long as they're used with stereo headphones. Of course you'd need at least one download for each of Beta, Alpha, Theta and Delta.

So, is your brain keeping you awake when you want to sleep, or do you want to sleep when you should be up and active? There are many indications that you might be out of balance, and bearing in mind that such imbalances have the potential to create emotional and neuro-physical problems, perhaps this is an area that warrants consideration.

CHAPTER EIGHTEEN

Medicinal Herbs and Spices

'Ounce for ounce, herbs and spices have more antioxidants than any other food group.'
– Michael Greger

I'm no expert on this subject, so if you're hoping for an encyclopaedic chapter, I'm afraid I'll disappoint you, and can only suggest that you get hold of a book like, for example, 'The Complete Guide to Herbs & Spices' by Nancy J Hajeski. However, I did learn a little about the medicinal value of these plants during my journey, and in this chapter, I'd like to briefly cover those I found, and continue to find, helpful.

Herbs and spices are available in several guises. For cooking purposes, you can of course buy most of them in their raw state, you can even grow them yourself. These are not as medicinally powerful as some of the other options, but they do have antioxidant qualities and they do enhance the flavour of your food.

The other main options are -

1) Teas, which are easy to prepare and do have benefits.

2) Tinctures, which I feel are the most powerful option medicinally, but also the most expensive.

3) In powder form, which after comparing, cost, efficacy and convenience became my choice.

You can also buy most herb powders ready encapsulated, but in my experience a good part of the capsule tends to be taken up with anti-caking agents, bulking agents and preservatives, though to be fair, the preservatives used are often natural ones, like vitamin C in the form of ascorbic acid, for example. But this isn't an option I'd recommend, though that's just my opinion. Anyway, buying the powders and filling your own capsules is so much cheaper than buying them ready made, and you avoid the additives.

Here in the UK, my preferred suppliers are – Superfood World, who have a quite limited range, but all their offerings are one hundred percent organic and of very high quality. Indigo Herbs, who have a huge range of teas, tinctures and powders, some organic and some not, that are good quality, and their customer service is excellent. Amazon also offer a good range, but most of the providers are unfamiliar to me, though of course that doesn't make them bad.

I add some of my powders to my daily smoothie, which I discuss in another chapter. But mostly, I encapsulate them myself. I do this using a small, inexpensive capsule machine, which is creatively called 'the capsule machine'. It produces twenty-four capsules at a time and the process takes about ten minutes. The capsules (size 00) cost about one penny each if you buy a pack of one thousand. I find this approach to be cheap and convenient. Amazon sell the machine and the capsules.

So which herbs and spices do I use and what are their benefits? In total I keep fourteen readily to hand. I take some on a daily basis and others as and when. The fourteen are, in no particular order –

Rhodiola Rosea – This is an adaptogen, meaning that it helps rebalance any imbalance in the body. It's especially useful in increasing energy, reducing fatigue, dampening the stress hormone cortisol, increasing brain function and reducing depression. I use it in capsules on a now and then basis, relying on intuition to tell me when.

Turmeric – This is a mild antidepressant, it has the potential to reduce the formation of blood clots, it can help heal wounds, it's a worthwhile adjunct to cancer treatment, and it helps with blood sugar control. However, I use it daily as a really good anti-inflammatory. Before I developed an interest in herbs and spices, I had an arthritic left-hand forefinger and a creaky and sometimes painful, left knee. They are no more, and I thank turmeric for that. I mix it with black pepper, which increases absorption quite dramatically, in a ratio of eighty percent turmeric to twenty percent black pepper. I add a small teaspoon of this combination to my daily smoothie.

Schisandra – This reduces inflammation, supports adrenal function, improves liver function, improves mental function and mildly improves sexual function. I take it in capsules when intuition tells me to.

Saw Palmetto – About sixteen years ago, I had part of my prostate gland removed, something I wouldn't have done knowing what I know now. At the time, I was told the operation would need to be repeated in around five years, then at similar intervals going forward. I take two capsules a day of saw palmetto and nettle root, combined in a 50/50 ratio. Those further operations never happened and my prostate gland is fine.

Milk Thistle – This has anti-cancer properties, it may help control blood sugar, and is anti-aging, But above all, it's a really good liver detoxifier. I don't use it every day now, but I do use it quite regularly. When I do, I take two capsules a day.

Cayenne Pepper – This helps digestion, it can relieve some migraines, it reduces blood clot formation, it's good for joints and nerves, it's anti-inflammatory, and anti-fungal. I take two capsules a day, one before each main meal.

Cinnamon – This is very high in antioxidants, it's anti-inflammatory, it supports heart function, it helps stabilize blood sugar, it enhances brain function and it is antiviral and antifungal. I add a large teaspoon to my daily smoothie. Important note – It is important to use only Ceylon cinnamon, NOT cassia cinnamon, which can be toxic in large doses.

Ashwagandha – This is another adaptogen that brings balance throughout the body. It improves underactive thyroid function, benefits adrenal fatigue, combats stress, anxiety and depression, balances blood sugar levels, boosts immune function, increases stamina and muscle strength and improves sexual function. I used this daily for a long time, taking two capsules a day. I still use it when intuition tells me to.

Black pepper – This has potential anti-cancer properties, it protects the liver, it's anti-inflammatory and anti-bacterial, it helps digestion and brain health, and may lower blood pressure in some cases. I use it mixed with turmeric. See above.

Moringa – This is higher than average in antioxidants, it is anti-inflammatory, it balances hormones, it aids digestion, it balances blood sugar levels and improves brain health. I take this as and when, based on intuition.

Astragalus – This is another adaptogen that offers many benefits. It's anti-inflammatory, it's a great immune booster that can slow tumour growth, it's heart healthy, it helps minimise diabetes complications, it's a fairly strong antioxidant, and it helps alleviate chemotherapy side effects. I used a lot of this at one point, but now, I use it from time to time.

Ginger – This is great for digestion, but it also relieves nausea, is anti-fungal, has cancer prevention properties, helps regulate blood sugar levels, and relieves stiff muscles and joints

I take two capsules a day. I also use it in a morning lemon drink that I describe in my breakfast chapter.

Nettle root – As mentioned above, I use this with saw palmetto for prostate health.

Amla – Also known as Indian gooseberry. This offers good liver support, it has anti-cancer properties, it's anti-inflammatory, it benefits hair and skin, it aids digestion and improves cognitive function. I did use it extensively in the past, but not so often now – as and when.

These descriptions are necessarily brief. For much greater in-depth descriptions of herb/spice benefits, including but not restricted to the above, I'd suggest a visit to droxe.com, which is a very good website for all manner of medical information. Just enter any herb/spice that interests you into the site's search box.

In summary, getting to know something about the medicinal properties of herbs and spices does involve a fair bit of research, but in my experience, such research has the potential to provide you with many health benefits. For example, you may have noticed that several of the above, especially turmeric, have anti-inflammatory properties, and inflammation is a major feature of every chronic illness I know of.

CHAPTER NINETEEN

Essential Oils

'It doesn't get much greener than essential oils: when used correctly, they are among Mother Nature's most potent remedies.'
- Amy Leigh Mercree,

I'm a believer in the medicinal properties of herbs and spices, but if anything, I'm an even greater believer in the medicinal properties of essential oils, which quite dramatically amplify the healing potential of the plants from which they're derived.

To most people, essential oils are what aromatherapists use, perhaps when giving you a nice massage. That's true, but they're so much more than that. They can be used in a diffuser to create wonderful health-giving aromas throughout your home. They can be applied to the skin, almost always with a carrier oil for dilution, for relaxation or to target any number of health issues. For go anywhere convenience, they can be inhaled, either from the bottle or from specially designed inhalers. They can be blended to supply numerous benefits, the particular blend depending on your objective. In some cases they can be taken internally, to aid digestion, to target particular organ complaints, or as a more direct attack on some infection or other. Diffusers, carrier oils and inhalers are widely available. Amazon carry a wide variety.

However, and this is very important, because of their high potency, there are risks and dangers associated with some oils if not used correctly. Therefore, unless your objective is very simple, to create a nice smell around your home, for example, I think it's essential to read and absorb at least one comprehensive and expertly written book on the subject. I'll make three recommendations at the end of this chapter.

Then there is the question of quality, and quality is the key issue when buying oils other than for the most-simple uses, and even then, poor quality can create problems.

Because of the rising interest in essential oil usage, a bandwagon has developed, and there are now numerous spurious manufacturers and providers. Some oils are chemically rather than plant derived. Some are diluted and/or have unwanted additives, which renders them useless. Some contain impurities that can have negative effects on your mind and body. Some are just plain fakes. And some are sold by the multi-level marketing route. These may or may not be good quality, but because of the numerous tiers of people taking a cut, they're invariably over-priced. After trying many makes here in the UK, I now use just three, which one depending on the proposed usage. These are –

nhrorganicoils.com. I'd suggest that these might well be the best organic oils in the world. They're certainly super clean and correctly derived from the best organic plants. However, as is usually the case with 'the best', they're probably the most expensive. If I were rich, I'd use this company exclusively. But I'm not rich.

Evolutionorganics.com. I use this company a lot for various products, but here we're talking about essential oils. They carry two ranges, Dr Mercola and Organixx, both of which are pure, correctly derived and organic. I wouldn't put them quite up there with NHR, but they're close and quite a lot cheaper. I'm happy to use them for the vast majority of my needs.

indigo-herbs.co.uk. Their range is pure and correctly derived, but not organic. I use these when the highest quality isn't essential. They're very competitively priced.

Along with a few carrier oils, though I mainly use fractionated coconut oil as a carrier, I keep a personal stock of around forty different essential oils, and it wouldn't be practical to discuss them all in a book like this. But to give you a flavour of what essential oils can do, the following are the ten that I use most frequently, and I'd suggest that if you're interested in exploring essential oils further, a selection from these ten would make a good starter kit.

Lavender. Amongst other things, this is an amazingly useful sleep aid, it soothes burns and cuts, it's a good anxiety reliever, in some cases it can reduce blood pressure, it can help balance blood sugar in some cases, it can improve skin health and can be a useful aid in relieving tension headaches and migraines.

Peppermint. Amongst other things, this is a good muscle relaxant, it helps relieve respiratory conditions, it can improve energy, applied to the temples it can ease headaches, it's a very good digestive aid, and it's a great addition to home-made toothpaste and mouthwash.

Eucalyptus. Amongst other things, this is great for lung infections, it can alleviate asthma and allergy symptoms, it can help with shingles, it aids with wound care and can improve energy and focus.

Lemon. Amongst other things, this promotes lymphatic drainage, it helps clear mucus, it helps support the gallbladder, it's an immune booster, it's a good multi-surface cleaner, and it can reduce allergy symptoms.

Rosemary. Amongst other things, this is anti-inflammatory, it can improve cognitive performance, it can help regulate blood sugar levels, it has pain reduction properties, it improves liver and gallbladder function, it can help ease respiratory complaints and it's a useful addition to a detoxification regime.

Tea Tree. Amongst other things, this is an insect repellent, it's a great antiseptic for cuts and scrapes, it's anti-viral, anti-bacterial, anti-fungal and anti-mold, and it's a good addition to homemade soap and shampoo.

Frankincense. This is the most expensive of my oils, but has many properties including anti-tumour potential, it can help with Alzheimer's disease, it boosts the immune system, it helps reduce inflammation, it can combat stress and negative emotions, it can improve ageing skin and it encourages healthy hormone levels.

Clove. Amongst other things, this is a brilliant toothache reliever, it can improve blood circulation, it's a good insect repellent, it's a good muscle and joint pain reliever. It can help with ear ache, and it helps clean the blood.

Geranium. Amongst other things, this promotes youthful skin, it helps balance hormones, it's a kidney cleanser, it can reduce the appearance of Eczema and it's a good wound healer.

Fir Needle. Amongst other things, this helps with respiratory issues, it has anti-tumour properties, it's a pain reliever, it's a good sanitizer, and it may be helpful in the treatment of Osteoporosis.

For the methodology of using the above for the purposes mentioned, see the previously promised book recommendations below, especially the first one.

Book recommendations

'Essential oils, ancient medicine' by Dr Josh Axe, Ty Bollinger and Jordan Rubin. This does have some religious connotations, but it provides lots of useful background and 'how to use safely' information. It contains lots of detail on around fifty oils, including carrier oils, and many pages on treating numerous conditions, and on making your own household, personal care and oral care products. Although I feel these three books complement each other well, if I were buying just one, this would be it.

'The directory of essential oils' by Wanda Sellar. This is a really good reference book. It has very little background information, but brilliantly detailed information on eighty oils, including what each one can be helpful for medicinally. I refer to this book regularly to refresh my memory.

'The healing power of essential oils' by Eric Zielinski, D.C. Another really useful reference book. Yes, this one also has religious connotations, but it includes useful guides on essential oil use, and recommendations for nearly every occasion along with all manner of useful tips and general information.

If you'd like to become really knowledgeable about the many uses of essential oils, I feel this threesome in combination will tell you everything you'll ever need to know.

Finally, please do keep in mind that this chapter is just a simple introduction to the huge subject of essential oils, and it would be unwise to dive into them based only on what I've written here. Remember, essential oils can cause harm if not used properly, so please get well informed.

CHAPTER TWENTY

Toxicity

'The governments weaponize toxins that the masses are routinely exposed to, and then denies the known toxicity of them.' – **Steven Magee**

'If you are in a toxic environment, you will waste away.' – **Richie Norton**

We live in a toxic world, and many of the toxins we're exposed to are unavoidable or at least very difficult to avoid. We shouldn't worry too much about those because as we can't do anything about them, the worrying will create stress, and stress is yet another major toxin adding to the load.

However, there are toxins that we can do something about if we're mindful to, and reducing or even eliminating these will substantially reduce the load on our digestion and detoxification organs–the liver, kidneys, colon, lungs, and skin, and our lymph system, freeing up energy that can be used by our immune system and our healing mechanisms, making it much easier to regain our health.

In the diet and water chapters, I talked about reducing the toxins we put in our bodies. Here, I'd like to talk about some of the toxins in our homes and those we put on our bodies because, these, as with those reduced or eliminated via what we eat and drink, we can also do something about.

In our homes

Air fresheners, whether sprays, freestanding or plug-ins are all highly toxic. What's the alternative? An easy one is essential oils used in a diffuser. There are plenty of reasonably priced diffusers available on Amazon and elsewhere, and you can use any essential oil of your choice. Geranium is quite nice, but there are many other possibilities, depending on your personal taste. When buying essential oils though, check the label and buy only those that have no other ingredients. Another option is to regularly brew coffee or bake bread, both of which create great smells.

Household cleaning products. Most of the mainstream products are toxic, though the ecover range and a few others are okay to use. Alternatively, consider using things like steam cleaners, white vinegar, lemon, baking soda and food grade hydrogen peroxide. There is plenty of information on the internet regarding how to use these.

What you put on your body

If you lie in the bath for half an hour, the water in the bath will have reduced by around a pint, and I'm not including the water still on you when you get out of the bath. Where did it go? You sucked it in via your skin. I mention this to illustrate that some of everything you put on your skin is absorbed, eventually getting into your blood stream, and much of what you put on your skin is toxic, and you don't want it getting into your bloodstream, from where it has access to every cell in your body. The following are examples.

Hair spray. Try spraying this on your hand then feel it. It's sticky goo, and every time you spray your hair, some of that sticky goo ends up in your lungs, and I'd put that sticky goo up there with smoking in terms of toxicity. Some people in the natural world suggest making your own with water, sugar and essential oils, but I've been given to understand that this approach doesn't work very well. That understanding could be wrong, but I suspect not. So I'm afraid I don't know of a well proven viable alternative. If you really must use hair spray, I'd suggest doing so in an open space, holding your breath, pinching your nose and closing your eyes, which are super toxin absorbers.

Talcum powder. This is carcinogenic, and as you use it, you breathe it in. So I would never use it.

Hand, face and body creams. In general, these are toxic, and the more expensive they are, the more toxic they seem to be. That's based on my experience of reading labels. Even most baby lotions contain a worrying array of chemicals. As alternatives, consider organic coconut oil, either the normal type or the fractionated type, which is liquid at room temperature. Both are a little greasy, and if you use too much you won't like it, so don't use too much. If required, essential oils can be added for fragrance. With the fractionated coconut oil, just a few drops are all you need. Organic aloe vera gel, Argan oil and shea butters are good, too. I make my own moisturiser – see end of chapter.

Perfumes. These are super toxins. As an alternative, try experimenting with good quality essential oils.

Cosmetics. These are very toxic, and I'm afraid that includes the current trend for fancy nail colouring, which contains chemicals like formaldehyde, toluene, DBP and TPHP, which have been connected to cancer, autoimmunity and hormone disruption. Personally, I'd say grow old naturally, but knowing that wouldn't go down well with many, I'd suggest you research the growing number of organic, chemical free cosmetic companies. So maybe discuss the possibilities with Mr Google. But if you can't bear the thought of not using your favourite brand, at least check the ingredients and google anything that you're not familiar with. You might be shocked by what you find.

Hair dye. Major brands are one of the most toxic things you can put on your body. But, again, there are natural alternatives, so while you're consulting Mr Google about cosmetics, why not ask him about clean hair dyes, too?

Antiperspirants and deodorant. Both are toxic and they're usually applied right where some major lymph nodes are, and that seriously concerns me. Unless you have some sort of excess sweating issue, I'd avoid antiperspirants completely because sweating is a great way to detoxify, and that's good. And please don't be fooled by the 'stone' type deodorants. Most if not all of them contain aluminium, which is a powerful neurotoxin. This fact is usually disguised by putting 'alum' on the ingredient label in tiny print. Alternative – see end of chapter.

Toothpaste. Most are full of nasty chemicals including fluoride, which is a toxic by-product of fertilizer production and/or an industrial waste product of the aluminium smelting industry. Yes there are sometimes tiny amounts of natural fluoride in water and some foods, but they're not the same thing at all. And you don't need fluoride to keep your teeth healthy. There are some fairly 'clean' toothpastes out there, but they tend to be very expensive. Alternatives – see end of chapter.

Mouthwash. Again, most contain chemicals your body doesn't like, and swishing in the mouth results in almost instant absorption into the bloodstream. Alternative – see end of chapter.

Showers and baths. First, your body's skin is heavily populated by beneficial bacteria, and every time you wash your skin, a few of them go to bacteria heaven. I'm not suggesting that you should get smelly, but it is possible to be over-clean.

Right, to business: unless you have a whole house water filtration system, part of what you're absorbing into your body is toxicity from the water you bathe in. There's little you can do about many of the toxins involved, but there is one that you can neutralise, and it's a biggie. Chlorine. I shower, and I use a vitamin C shower head. There are several options available on Amazon and elsewhere. It neutralises almost all of the chlorine via a vitamin C filter. Filters last me about three months and are reasonably cheap and easy to replace. If you prefer a bath, adding a dessert spoon of cheap ascorbic acid will do what my shower head does. I've heard that Borax added to bath water can neutralise fluoride. I've never been able to verify that to my satisfaction, but trying it will do no harm.

Soap, shower gel and shampoo. Most major brands contain an array of toxins. Alternative – see end of chapter.

Electromagnet fields (EMFs). You don't see them in your home, but they permeate it. You don't put them in or on your body, but they certainly disrupt the body's own magnetic field, and in a few people, that can be catastrophic, leaving them bed bound for life. Many more people experience things like headaches and sleeplessness, not realising that the cause is a disrupted personal magnetic field.

Fortunately, most people don't have symptoms caused by EMFs, but if they can devastate a few people's lives and create relatively mild symptoms in more people, I'd suggest that it's possible that in thirty or forty years-time exposure to these fields might be considered as dangerous as a twenty-a-day smoking habit. Remember, that for many years during the mid- nineteen-hundreds, doctors recommended cigarettes for chest ailments and as a general health aid. So when authorities tell you that EMFs are harmless, can you really be sure that they're right? Following a great deal of research, I'm convinced that they're not.

At the time of writing, 5G isn't far away, and by the time you read this, it will probably be here. Great, faster broadband and better mobile connections. But consider this, which I came across recently –

'More than two hundred and thirty scientists and doctors from forty countries recently appealed to the

World Health Organisation calling for a moratorium of 5G wireless technology, stating that the 5G wireless signal should be moved from Group 2B carcinogen categorisation to Group 1, the same as asbestos and arsenic.'

We can't escape EMFs because they're everywhere, but there are a few ways to reduce exposure to them –

If you haven't already got a smart meter, don't be talked into having one. They're not necessary and they emit very powerful EMFs throughout your home, even when they're in a box on an outside wall.

If you have a laptop, don't have it on your lap. Hold it as far away from your body as you can.

Don't hold your mobile phone close to your head, use speaker phone, and where possible, don't keep it in a pocket without switching it off. Keep calls short, text instead.

Switch your WIFI off whenever it's not in use. If you can't do that, at least switch it off during sleeping hours.

There are more and more WIFI household appliances becoming available. Don't buy them.

It's easy to believe that you've been putting what I've described as toxins on your body and in your mouth for years and they haven't harmed you. As far as I know, there's nothing in the medical literature called 'toxin disease', but I'm quite sure that many of the diseases of aging like heart disease, cancer, diabetes and arthritis etc, are at least in part caused by toxins. But if you finish up with such a disease, you won't relate it to the toxic substances you've been using because, as I said, you've been using them for years with no apparent ill effects. The body's detox systems, liver, kidneys, colon, skin, lungs and lymph system, are pretty good at eliminating toxins on a daily basis, but over time, possibly decades, they get overwhelmed, and when that happens your body starts to deteriorate. Then, one day, you lose your health. Perhaps because you dyed your hair, for example, for forty years. Who's to say?

I hope this chapter hasn't been too dispiriting. If it has then please bear in mind that although it's impossible for most people to avoid all toxins, if you eat healthily, drink healthy water, minimise the use of toxic products in your home and on your body, and minimise your EMF exposure as best you can, you'll be way ahead of the vast majority of the population. Remember, your body can deal with a great deal of toxic exposure. It's not until the load becomes overwhelming that the problems start. Generally, do your best, and, hopefully, you might well avoid the tipping point.

My personal care products

Moisturiser. Three quarters fill a 50ml brown or blue glass jar with aloe vera gel, add a teaspoon of Argan oil and a quarter teaspoon of colloidal silver. Mix well. You only need a very small amount and it sinks into the skin very quickly. The 50ml jar will last for ages.

Deodorant. I make this in 500ml batches, putting the finished product into ten 50ml brown or blue glass jars. To 500ml of fractionated coconut oil (the liquid form), add a dessert spoon of aluminium free baking soda. Add forty to fifty drops of essential oil. I use ten drops of cypress and forty drops of sandalwood. Options more appealing to ladies are probably lavender, lemon, ylang ylang and jasmine, either singular to your preference or combined. A bit of experimentation is advised. Mix well and pour into the 50ml jars. The mixture will separate in the jars, but a good shake is all that's needed. Apply with clean fingers, using small amounts wherever needed.

Toothpaste. I make this in 250ml batches, then put into 50ml brown or blue glass jars. To 250ml of fractionated coconut oil, add ten drops of tea tree oil, ten drops of clove oil and thirty to forty drops of peppermint oil. Mix well, then add equal amounts of aluminium free baking soda and diatomaceous earth to get the consistency you want. I get it to a thick paste. This isn't the best tasting toothpaste in the world, but it's palatable, it works brilliantly, and whatever is absorbed in to your bloodstream is good for you.

Mouthwash. I use a 300ml bottle simply because that's what I had to hand when I first started making it. Fill the bottle with pure water, as pure as you can get, then add 1 drop of basil essential oil, 1 drop of tea tree oil, one drop of clove oil and four drops of peppermint oil. Shake the bottle before each use. Swish in the mouth for thirty seconds to a minute.

Washing. For my hair, I use Dr Mercola volumizing shampoo. This is quite expensive, so for a lower cost option Faith In Nature offer a wide range of shampoos and shower gels that are pretty clean. For everything else, I use Dr Bronner's baby mild pure organic castile soap. I don't, but if you want to you can add an essential oil of your choice for fragrance.

All the ingredients of the above are readily available, but I'd advise using organic options wherever possible. This applies especially to essential oils. Also, before using any essential oil rub a drop mixed with three of four of drops of carrier oil – coconut or olive oil are fine – on to your inner arm or other sensitive areas and leave for ten minutes. If no skin reaction occurs, it should be fine for you. But stop use if a reaction occurs in the future. Such reactions aren't usual, but they can happen to some people.

Finally, most of the above-mentioned ingredients don't like the light, and that's the reason for using brown or blue glass jars.

PART THREE

Mental Considerations

Chapter 21 – The importance of belief in the power of belief

Chapter 22 – Mind programmes and genetics

Chapter 23 – Acceptance, forgiveness and letting go

Chapter 24 – Stress, anxiety and panic attacks

Chapter 25 – Mindfulness

Chapter 26 – Visualisation and affirmations

CHAPTER TWENTY-ONE

The Importance Of Belief In The Power Of Belief

'You have to believe. Otherwise, it will never happen.' – **Neil Gaiman**

'Your belief determines your action and your action determines your results, but first you have to believe.' – **Mark Victor Hansen**

'If I have the belief that I can do it, I shall surely acquire the capacity to do it even if I may not have it at the beginning.' – **Mahatma Gandhi**

To my mind, belief in the power of belief is the most important non-physical part of recovering your health. I hold the view that you must believe that you'll get well, deep down. Not 'want to', not 'hope so', but 'know so', because a firm belief inspires determination and determination is what gets you where you want to go.

At this stage, I'd like to stress that belief at the very deepest level isn't the same as what many people incorrectly think of as positive thinking when they attempt to convince themselves that something that is, isn't. The mistake they make is in using mantras that emphasise the 'isn't'. For instance, 'I can be a success'. This tells the subconscious mind that you're not a success because the subconscious 'thinks' logically, so 'I can be' means 'I'm not'. The subconscious then puts in place mechanisms that keep you unsuccessful because it 'think's that's what you want. The point here is that a sick person isn't going to get well using mantras that emphasise the sickness.

So, does true, deep down belief really have a phenomenal power that can change things and solve major problems? Can it be instrumental in driving you towards recovery? Well I'm convinced that it can, and via a short story then a simple fact, I'm hoping to convey why.

The story

I've read numerous verifiable stories demonstrating the power of belief, but this is one that I've heard from several sources, including from one of the participants, Lynne McTaggart, a respected investigative journalist who has concentrated her efforts on health issues and medical treatments, both conventional and alternative, for several decades.

Some years back, her mother-in-law developed a problem with her breast. Being a sensitive and private lady, she kept this to herself for a very long time. Eventually, in Lynne McTaggart's words, her breast resembled a piece of raw meat, and at last, she sought medical advice. She was quickly referred to an oncologist who conferred with several colleagues, all of whom agreed that she was beyond medical help and would be dead within three or four months.

Lynne McTaggart then took her mother-in-law to see

Dr Patrick Kingsley, a private practice doctor, now retired, who successfully specialised in the treatment of cancer and MS, generally involving unconventional methods. He examined the breast, smiled, then gently said in a reassuring tone, 'Oh yes, I'm sure we can deal with that.' Within a few months, the cancer was gone and the breast was healed.

Lynne McTaggart, and remember, she's a respected investigative journalist, believes that it was those few words that saved her mother-in-law's life as much as or more than the mainly unconventional treatment that followed. She had been subject to well over a year of concealed fear, followed by a dire prognosis from several oncologists. Then this one man with his confident smile and strong reassurances, gave her hope that was powerful enough to instil belief.

The fact

There's actually a great deal of scientific evidence confirming the power of belief, but I use the following because I feel it's both simple and unarguable.

Pharmaceutical companies tend to concentrate their efforts on relief from symptoms rather than cures. When they create a new drug that they believe will relieve a specific set of symptoms related to a particular illness, they usually arrange a randomized, double-blind, placebo-controlled trial, involving X number of sufferers of that illness, half of whom will receive the new drug and half of whom will receive a placebo, or sugar pill. Nobody, including those carrying out the trial, knows which participants have received the new drug and which have received the placebo. All this is to confirm that the pharmaceutical company's belief in the new drug's efficacy was justified.

Typically, between twenty percent and forty percent of those taking the placebo will see their symptoms improve or completely resolve. If the actual drug achieves success by a few percentage points more than the placebo did, it is considered to be a success. I think it's generally accepted that very few, if any, drugs are anything like one hundred percent successful for everyone, in which case the difference between the placebo and drug results are often not that great.

Whatever, in clinical trials, many people are getting a degree of symptom relief from a simple sugar pill, a result that is often not much different to that produced by the drug. As the sugar pill has no medicinal value, to my mind, that's clear evidence that belief alone has a positive influence on the body's innate healing capability.

There are several ideas in other chapters of this book that might help in developing that power, and I'd suggest the visualisation and affirmations chapter as a suitable complement.

In my own case, it wasn't until I accepted that the medical system had failed me, that I began to believe I could help myself. It was then that things began to happen.

Finally, please be very aware that beliefs are beliefs, and negative beliefs are every bit as powerful as positive ones. So if you believe that your illness is for life, you'll almost certainly be right.

CHAPTER TWENTY-TWO

Mind Programmes And Genetic

'The function of the subconscious mind is to take your beliefs and turn them into reality'
– Dr Bruce Lipton

For most of my life I understood that the subconscious mind was the clever part. After all, people called it the creative mind. But it now seems that it's nothing more than a powerful computer, albeit a very useful one if its software works well. But for many, that's the problem, because we create our own software, and its quality depends very much on our thoughts, beliefs, desires and our environment.

Before we are born, the subconscious is pre-programmed to set up then monitor and adjust all the physical body's systems, thus ensuring that we can survive in the environment we're born into. Just imagine, for example, how impossible it would be to consciously keep your heart beating or your digestive system functioning efficiently. Other than that, though, it's a blank canvas waiting to be programmed, initially by our environment and our perceptions of our environment

For many decades, neurologists have known that the brain has four types of waveform, which are beta, alpha, theta and delta. A new born baby is in the brain state of theta, which is a mild hypnotic state. The baby remains in this state until around age seven, and this is why young children are such amazing learners, the degree of that learning capability being influenced by their environment. Just think about what, starting from scratch, a healthy seven-year-old has achieved. It really is truly amazing.

During this circa seven-year period children use imagery to establish programmes in their subconscious, one of the earliest of which will be the ability to crawl. At first, they will note that a particular limb movement translates to a changed position on the floor, and that's learned knowledge that they enjoy. Slowly, they realise that a combination of those limb movements creates greater movement across the floor. Initially they have to think about every movement of the crawling process, but gradually this thinking process diminishes, and eventually, they crawl without the need of conscious thought. A programme has been created.

By age seven, hundreds or even thousands of programmes have been installed, and these programmes will have a huge influence on the way their lives develop, and how their lives develop will depend on the quality of those programmes, which depend in turn on early environmental influences and their perception of those influences. In short, their future, including their future health, is broadly already defined, but not by divine intervention or anything else other than by themselves and their environment, which includes the people around them like parents, siblings, teachers, relatives and school friends etc.

So how important are these influences? Consider two children. One is brought up in a loving home, where the parents, read stories, arrange exciting trips and encourage learning in a loving way. They attend a good school and are taught by caring teachers. Their wider family are supportive and they have good schoolfriends. The other, though, exists in a home where the parents show little interest, where they're irritated by the child, where the child is disciplined in a cruel way. Their broader family are equally unsupportive, and they attend a school where they're mocked or bullied.

In both cases, programmes are being created. In the first case these programmes will be mainly positive, and the child will be confident and happy and, generally, they'll do well in all aspects of their future. In the second case, however, the reverse will be the case. By luck or good fortune, some may gradually overwrite the negative programmes that they've installed, perhaps moving on to great things, but most won't. They'll become carbon copies of their parents and they'll pass their own traits on to their children, not because of genes, but because of environment. So the quality of these early influences is extremely important.

A key thing to consider at this point is that your mind is around 5% conscious and 95% subconscious, and that your conscious mind is the creative part, creating thoughts, wishes and desires. It 'paints pictures' and converts these pictures in to chemistry. So, for example, if you feel under stress, you produce stress hormones, which may dramatically disrupt your body's balance. The subconscious constantly monitors what the conscious mind is creating and establishes programmes based on the repetitive and habitual messages it receives. The result of all this is that although the conscious mind is the creative part, the subconscious is in control most of the time, and it can and often does sabotage your health by installing self-created negative programmes.

It's important to understand that the conscious mind is busy just dealing with life around 95% of the time, so I'd like to ask you favour. Carefully monitor the thoughts that pop into your head for as long as you can without going bananas, which is usually about twenty minutes. You'll probably find that many, quite possibly most, of these thoughts will be negative, and such thoughts may eventually turn into reality via the programmes they install.

Based on what I've learned over the last few years, there is one programme that almost all of us have that I don't believe to be a good thing. Early in life we'll have observed several people getting ill, and we may have had some illness ourselves. And what do we learn to do? We go to the doctor. Having observed this several or, more probably, many times the subconscious creates a programme of 'if you're ill, you go to the doctor'.

Have you ever noticed that you book a doctor's appointment and that between setting off and arriving at the surgery you start to feel better? That's the 'illness programme' at work. Your subconscious has done its job and got you to the doctor's surgery, so it can then start the healing process, hence the starting to feel better.

Now I'm not suggesting that you should never consult a doctor, but I would suggest that maybe nine out of ten visits are unnecessary and potentially stressful, because given the right tools, the body can very often heal itself.

A quick example. Let's say you go to the doctor because you're a bit 'chesty'. The doctor listens to your chest, and with a serious expression asks you to spit into a container, saying he'll send the sample for testing. To be on the safe side, he then prescribes an antibiotic, saying that the test result will be back in seven days.

His serious expression concerns you. Could this be something serious? This thought creates anxiety, which reduces the function of your immune and digestive systems. By the time the test result is back, you're feeling fine so you assume the antibiotic has been effective. But the test result reveals that you had a viral infection rather than a bacterial one. So, the antibiotics had nothing to do with your recovery, but the strong placebo effect caused by your belief in the antibiotic probably supported your weakened immune system enabling it to get the job done. However, had you not gone to the doctor, it would probably have done the job alone and more quickly.

By age eight, children have moved out of theta, and are starting to establish programmes less influenced by those around them and more influenced by what they perceive to be going on in their world. These programmes might be good or bad, usually a combination of the two, but it's the pre-eight programmes that will most influence their future. If you're a parent with a young child, I think it's as well to bear that in mind.

What all this means is that every aspect of your life including health is controlled by your subconscious programmes, which can support your objectives or sabotage them. In many cases, they're heavily weighted towards the latter.

But what about genetic illness, illness inherited from previous generations? Surely, they're nothing to do with these programmes. Isn't it likely that your chronic illness is due to these genetics? The answer is that it is, in fact, very unlikely.

Genes are the blueprints used to manufacture the building blocks of cells. These building blocks are proteins, of which there are many, many types, and different cells require different proteins. It is your DNA's job to select the appropriate blueprint for the cell in which it resides. So, in effect, genes are the architect and DNA is the builder.

That was a huge oversimplification, but a fuller explanation is beyond the scope of this book, and the only point I'm aiming to make is that although genes are essential for our survival, they're not the key to solving everything that the Press intimated and continue to intimate when genetics became flavour of the month a few decades ago. If you'd like to study this subject further, I strongly recommend the work of Dr Bruce Lipton.

There is a widely held belief that if a gene turns itself off this will result in damage to corresponding cells because the DNA loses its blueprint, and this can lead to cancer, for example. In fact, many early researchers believed that genes had total control over our health.

Sadly, many women have had their breasts removed on discovering that they have the BRAC1 gene. It is true that this gene is genuinely related to the development of breast cancer, but the reality is that over fifty percent of the women who have this gene never develop breast cancer. So if this gene leads almost inevitably to cancer, as many will have you believe, why don't one hundred percent of the women who have it develop the disease?

Going back to the early research, many researchers did believe that if a gene turns itself off then a disease of some sort will follow, and that if they, the researchers, could switch it back on again, the disease could perhaps be cured.

But they were wrong in that because although genes can be and sometimes do get turned off, it's not the gene that's doing the turning. Epigenetics, which is the science of how the environment and our perception of the environment controls genetics, has demonstrated that you are not a victim of hereditary, you are the master of it, albeit unwittingly in most cases, because you can control your environment and your perceptions by sending signals to your cells via your nervous system, these signals having the ability to adjust the cell's behaviour.

For example, using the breast cancer gene again, if a woman's mother and grandmother had breast cancer and this woman hears about the breast cancer gene, she may perceive that she's destined for the same fate.

Well if she does what her mother and grandmother did, and holds the same beliefs that they had, she may well be right, because she'll create huge amounts of stress, which is understood to be a major potential cause of cancer. But it's she, or rather her subconscious programme, that unwittingly turned off the gene, not the gene itself.

If on the other hand, she understands and accepts the gene's potential but changes her thoughts and behaviour in a positive way then adjusts her environment and her perception of the risk, she's less likely to develop the cancer, meaning that the gene is not in control, she is.

I should say now that there are a few diseases that are inevitable because a specific gene is turned off or a specific piece of DNA is damaged. Two of these diseases, for example, are haemophilia and cystic fibrosis. But it's generally accepted that these particular genes or DNA pieces were faulty at conception or shortly after, and the resultant diseases are extremely rare, representing less than one percent of all known diseases.

So in summary, no, your genes most likely didn't switch themselves off and cause your illness, and illness and disease are rarely truly hereditary. Rather, it is our environment and our thoughts, beliefs and perceptions that influence our genetic health.

Okay, if we accept all that, what's to be done about faulty programming and misbehaving genes?

First, let's briefly recap. Our subconscious is programmed, and many of these programmes were installed before our eighth birthday and we are the programmers. The early programmes were created by our imagination, which in a young child's mind is more powerful than reality, and our internal and external environment, along with our perception of our environment. Also, thoughts of genetic possibilities might worry us when it comes to health.

What does all this mean?

What it means is that we are not victims, we arrived at where we are now via our own thoughts, desires, beliefs and environment. But if we don't like where we are now, we can change it, because we can control our thoughts, desires, beliefs and environment. We are in control. The question now is, how do we take that control and turn things around?

First, it's important to understand that not all of our programmes are bad. In fact, it's quite likely that most of them are good. Also, some are installed very quickly. For example, a child might burn its hand on a hot hob. Because the subconscious has protective instincts, it will install a programme almost instantly, ensuring that the child will be very wary of hobs in the future.

Others though, can take a long time to install because, other than when urgency is required, the subconscious programmes are established by habit and habits take time to form. How long did it take you to learn to drive without thinking about where the clutch is or how much to turn the steering wheel to negotiate a corner? For this reason, new long-term habits have to be established to overwrite the old programmes, and this can take several weeks of persistence to achieve – so patience is needed.

Before we go further into that, some people have the determination, will and patience to deal with this issue themselves, but others don't, and they will most likely give up way before they can reasonably expect to see results. These people are likely to benefit from professional help, which if provided properly, can often work more quickly than the do-it-yourself approach.

In my experience, though, mainstream allopathic medicine has no idea how to supply such help, so my suggestion would be to seek out an energy healing practitioner. There are many varieties of energy healing, but three that I particularly respect are –

1) The Emotion Code, which I used myself and will write further on in another chapter.

2) Psych-K.

3) Emotional Freedom technique (EFT).

You'll find local practitioners of these modalities by consulting Mr Google, but unfortunately, as is the case with most professions, some practitioners are good at what they do and others aren't. If you make contact with one, make it clear that you're looking to overwrite subconscious negative programmes. If it's obvious that they don't know what you mean, move on. Finally, another viable option might be to seek out a really good hypnotherapist, but the same question should be asked.

So, back to the DIY option, keeping in mind the need

for determination, will, intention and patience, I think affirmations are a great way forward because they involve constant repetition and constant repetition creates habits and, over time, these habits can overwrite programmes created by previous habits.

I've known people who despite starting off enthusiastically, gave up on affirmations too soon. This was simply because they incorrectly anticipated quick results, underestimating the time taken to establish new habits. So it's very important to understand the importance of a few things that are required for affirmations to become effective.

1) You need the ability to clear your mind. If this is a problem for you, mindfulness practice, which I'll touch on in another chapter, is a good way to develop the necessary skill.

2) You need to have a strong intent, which is a clear idea of what you're aiming to achieve and the determination to achieve it.

3) You need to develop a strong belief in what you're doing.

4) You need to be really persistent when nothing seems to be happening, and you are very likely to experience periods, possibly long ones, when 'nothing is happening'.

How will you know when you've got it right? During a successful affirmation, without realising it you'll almost certainly develop a contented smile. When that happens, you're on the right track.

This book is about recovering good health, so what would be an appropriate affirmation for that?

The one I wrote and used before sleep and on waking is -

'I have good health and wellbeing, mentally, physically, emotionally and spiritually. All four aspects of my being work symbiotically and in harmony for equal benefit to all, ensuring long term continuation of my good health and wellbeing.'

If you're comfortable with that, then by all means use it, but anything that you come up with yourself will be effective as long as you're basically saying the same thing.

Doing this before sleep and on waking are important, because that's when your dominant brain wave pattern tends to be theta, and theta is the pattern most conducive to acceptance of your instruction by your subconscious. However, habits are created by repetition, and there's nothing wrong with repeating your affirmation at other times when you're in a calm and relaxed state.

When I started with affirmations, I had a problem in that I'd think, 'I'm saying I'm healthy but I know I'm not, so I'm just trying to kid myself.' But I eventually learned that I wasn't.

Affirmations are about energy and specifically about the energy of intent. What you're actually doing is writing an energy blueprint of your intention. A house can't be built without plans, the blueprint, but once the builder has the blueprint, he can envisage the house, and can then build it. Without the blueprint, the plot of land would stay as it is. Everything man has ever created started with a thought, and thought is energy. Without those thoughts, nothing manmade would exist. So you're not kidding yourself, you're designing your future. When the affirmation is made, what you've affirmed does exist energetically as a blueprint with which your subconscious can start work because it has a clear picture of what's required at the material level and the programme overwrite can begin.

So to reiterate, it's crucially important to understand the key point, which is that affirmations must state your objective as though it already exists, because at the energy level, it does. And you must be precise. If, for example, you were to say, 'I am getting better...' What does that convey to your subconscious? It might wonder how much better you want to get? Your subconscious only understands thoughts or words that convey a status of 'existing now'. It requires specific instructions, not vagaries.

Okay, but what if I'm concerned about genetics and my family history? The same principles apply. Only you can switch a gene on or off and you do that with your thoughts, beliefs, desires and perceptions, so change them. If you've already switched a gene off, that's a programme. Overwrite it with the help of affirmations.

I do hope that I've conveyed the importance of mind programmes and genetics here, because I believe that getting to grips with the information in this chapter represents an extremely important step on the road to recovery.

A footnote on lifespan –

Depending on what research you read, we as organisms have the capacity to live for one hundred and twenty years, or one hundred and forty years or beyond. So why don't we?

We are taught from childhood that we die at around age seventy or eighty or ninety, and as we grow up, we see our grandparents, parents and others do just that. So we develop a programme in our subconscious to do the same. The need then, is to replace that programme with one that agrees with the research, and stop counting birthdays. I suspect that after we get to around age forty, we may at the subconscious level be counting each birthday as a step closer to death, and I don't see that as a good thing to do.

A question that has intrigued me and that I'd urge you to dwell on is -

'How old would you be if you didn't know how old you are?'

CHAPTER TWENTY-THREE

Acceptance, Forgiveness And Letting Go

"The truth is, unless you let go, unless you forgive yourself, unless you forgive the situation unless you realise that the situation is over, you cannot move forward" – **Steve Maraboli**

The Hawaiian system called Ho'oponoopano helps change your thoughts and how you relate to things in a very simple way. In essence, it is to repeat four thoughts whenever you feel uncomfortable or unhappy in any way, and also when you think of anything negative in your past. These thoughts will help you release the old programming that has been built in and therefore will change the experiences for the better. They will initially work on your own personal subconscious beliefs and patterning, then with the resonance you have with others and the wider field of energies around you, all of which are influencing you. You say them even if you have a difficulty that you feel is none of your making, as it will resolve the negative energy of the situation and people's attitudes to you will change as well as the situations you find you are in.

The statements are:

I am sorry

Please forgive me
Thank you
I love you

Say them several times every day in connection with any aspects of life that you feel are unsatisfactory at the moment and any other times that you feel less than blissful. As you focus on these statements you can feel the energies being transmuted to love and feel the hard resistance dissolving.

The 'I am sorry' is to apologise to yourself for holding on to things that are hurting you and making life difficult.

The 'Please forgive me' is to ask the Universe to transmute the negative patterns to love.

The 'Thank you' is the acceptance of the change from negativity to love.

And the 'I love you' is to the forces that have helped you to change. It is not that God or the Universe needs to hear it; it is that YOU need to hear it.

The above isn't from me, it was given to me by an amazing energy healer called Jay Cubitt. But it's here because this ancient Hawaiian philosophy has some similarities to what this section is about. I thought, therefore, that it makes sense to read them in conjunction with each other, perhaps gaining something from each.

If 'mind' is hurt, and I believe that in pretty much all

illness, physical or mental, it is, then it's an emotional issue. The emotions involved are many, and in this context, all of them negative, hence the hurt, and they create destructive thoughts, often subconsciously, such as hate, revenge and condemnation.

Something or 'somethings' have happened in the past, often the distant past, perhaps as far back as the womb, that you don't necessarily dwell on consciously, but that fester and hurt 'mind', adversely affecting its interaction with the body resulting in physical damage. Very often, there is no conscious memory of the original event or events, but to get back on track, it or they must be addressed.

Some people will need professional assistance to deal with such deep-seated issues, but as long as they're comfortable with the concept that there's no particular need to establish exactly what the original cause or causes of hurt were, some people don't. Does it matter what they were? I don't think so. Is it necessary to know what caused an itch for a scratch to eliminate it? If you feel you have or might have issues, but can't accept this concept, then perhaps therapy is the answer. But if you can accept it, I believe there are three main things that need to worked on, which are acceptance, forgiveness and letting go.

Acceptance

To deal with the hurt, and doing so has a powerful potential to return 'mind's' ability to heal the body, you must first accept that such hurt exists. I don't know of anyone who hasn't been hurt by somebody at some time. If you think for a while, you'll probably come up with several personal examples, but if you don't, trust me, they exist, buried in your subconscious as a futile attempt to protect you. In fact, the ones you remember are least likely to be causing you harm. It's often the consciously forgotten ones that create major problems. So, the need is to accept that they exist, and that what they are doesn't really matter.

Forgiveness

This can be hard, but hopefully not too hard if you consider that those who hurt others have usually been hurt themselves and, therefore, have their own issues. As an extreme example, many child abusers were abused as a child themselves, meaning that they have a learned behaviour pattern that really isn't their fault. They do of course have to be prevented from causing harm, but, surely, they warrant a degree of sympathy for the misery they suffered, don't they? Not everyone is strong enough to shrug off their past and change for the better, but is weakness a valid reason for condemnation? And of course, many people cause hurt inadvertently, never realising what they have done.

Some people, though I suspect not many, might just be born bad. But if that's so, again, it's not their fault because you have no control over how you were born. We all have issues of some sort, and if someone's issues are powerful enough to cause them to hurt others, shouldn't we feel pity for them rather than hate or hostility?

But let's be selfish for a moment. Forgiveness isn't only

for those you need to forgive. In fact, they're unlikely to know that you've forgiven them. The forgiveness is also for you, and it's very important to understand that.

In whatever happened in the past, you had an involvement, and you might even have hurt the person who hurt you, perhaps unintentionally. It's crucial to forgive others, but it's equally crucial to forgive yourself. In fact many 'issues' are down to feelings of guilt, often a guilt that you don't know the source of. But the past is the past and you're no longer the person you were, so you must forgive yourself before you can move on.

In summary, the emotions created by being hurt just add further hurt, to you, not the perpetrator. So you don't need them, and a major key to dissolving them is forgiveness. Unless you can forgive the people who created those emotions in you, those emotions will remain and fester creating the imbalances that make you ill. The forgiveness is for your benefit, as much if not more than for those you are forgiving.

Letting go

What's the point in letting the past affect your here and now and your future? There is no point. Past happenings have no form or ability to hurt you unless you allow them to. Having mused on past hurt, whether consciously remembered or not, and forgiven others and yourself, you're in a position to release negative history as long as you're prepared to allow its release. So it's down to you. Just let it go.

In your own words, I think it's very powerful to have frequent conversations with yourself, at least daily until you feel a sense of release, along the lines of –

'I'm aware that I've allowed past hurts, those I remember and those that I don't, to adversely affect my present. I regret that and it must end so that my future can unfold free of issues. I've given thought to all those involved, those I remember and those that, consciously, I don't, and I now think of them in a spirit of love and forgiveness; I wish them well. For my own part, in order to move on as a better, happier and healthier person, I forgive myself for everything I've ever done that I wish I hadn't, remembered consciously or not. I now let go of all negative emotions because I no longer need them. My mind is now at ease.

But as I said, in your own words.

I thought long and hard before writing this because I'm very aware that many will reject the possibility that a hurt mind can result in a hurt body, and they may also reject the possible existence of their own deep rooted, well-hidden detrimental negative emotions. Furthermore, they may reject the approach described above as being nonsensical. And to be honest, it's not that long ago that I was in that camp, so I can hardly be critical of those opinions. But I hope that some might dwell a little on what's been said here because I'm convinced that acceptance, forgiveness and letting go are a crucially important element in releasing those parts of your past that hurt, and in doing so aid recovery from your physical imbalances.

Finally, whilst I believe that the above approach can be helpful for those who are comfortable with it, if you're not comfortable with it but feel that you have or might have emotional issues, psychotherapy or consultation with a skilled energy healer is likely be the best route to take.

CHAPTER TWENTY-FOUR

Stress, Anxiety And Panic Attacks

God grant me the serenity to accept the things I cannot change, the courage to change the things I can, and the wisdom to know the difference
— **Reinhold Niebuhr.**

Stress is what gets in the way of the future you want, whether that be good health or anything else. It precipitates all but around 1% of illness, that 1% being the true but very rare genetic diseases
— **Bruce Lipton.**

Before I say anything, I must willingly accept that what I do say in this chapter will be roundly condemned by the vast majority of GPs, counsellors, psychotherapists and psychiatrists. I accept their condemnation with good grace whilst at the same time suggesting that their cure rate when dealing with stress, anxiety and panic attacks really isn't that good, and I do mean cure rather than management or long-term medication.

So, what is stress? For my view in a nutshell, please see the Bruce Lipton quote above. But it's important to understand that there are two types of stress that need to be compared.

Good stress – this is a natural part of our physiology that was extremely useful to our ancient ancestors in an emergency. Picture paleo man happily going about his business when a predator appears and is charging towards him. The stress reflex automatically engages the autonomic nervous system, switching it from parasympathetic (the relaxed state) to sympathetic (the alert for danger state). This diverts blood away from the organs and the immune and digestive systems, to the muscles, especially those in his arms and legs. He can then react more quickly and more effectively to fight or flee, either killing the predator or escaping from it. This is called the fight or flight response. When the situation is resolved, the autonomic nervous system rebalances, stress evaporates, normal circulation resumes and he carries on happily with his business. In this situation, stress is extremely useful, perfectly normal and absolutely safe.

Bad stress – this is chronic stress. Nowadays we live in a stressful world, and of course if you have a chronic illness, that is stressful in itself. If we're chronically stressed, the physiological changes that we experience are exactly the same as those experienced by paleo man. But rather than settling down, they remain, resulting in long term diminished immune and digestive system function via a steady and persistent release of the stress hormones, Adrenalin, Norepinephrine and Cortisol, along with poor blood supply to the organs and, very likely, pain in the muscles and joints due to muscular tension. This can be extremely problematic because it can create a 'this is now normal' programme in the subconscious mind, so we often don't recognise that we're stressed. We then plough on, slowly creating a perfect storm for the development of all manner of physical harm.

So what is anxiety? I'd suggest that anxiety is simply the likely extension of chronic stress. You can have stress without anxiety but I don't think you can have anxiety without previously experiencing stress, and that previously experienced stress could be from the distant past, and consciously long forgotten. Left to their own devices, anxiety disorders can develop into panic attacks, which are an extreme version of anxiety and are horrendous things to experience.

Many people who have an anxiety disorder try to hide the fact, seemingly ashamed of their affliction. Well I have personal experience of these things and I'm not ashamed because they're simply an out-of-balance autonomic nervous system – a condition like any other condition. But fortunately, I believe that like the majority of conditions, they can be successfully resolved.

So if you have an anxiety disorder and/or suffer from panic attacks, and if you try to hide the fact from others or even yourself, STOP – they're nothing to be embarrassed about, and experiencing these things doesn't mean that you're a weak or pathetic person.

Talk to friends and family, explain how you're feeling but that you're working on dealing with it. I think you'll find this very liberating. Not only that, but being honest with others, and more importantly being honest with yourself, is a great first step towards recovery. And because displaying honesty takes courage, doing that alone demonstrates that you're not a weak or pathetic person, you're a strong person, and that strength will be an integral part of your recovery process.

So what can you do about stress, anxiety and panic attacks?

First, let's look at the medical system's approach. It usually prescribes medications like Prozac, Amitriptyline, Citalopram, Fluvoxamine etc, but your stress/anxiety wasn't caused by a deficiency of these chemicals so they are nothing more than symptom suppressors, and while ever you remain on them the underlying imbalance will remain. I should say that they may be helpful if taken for very short periods in severely acute situations, but in my opinion, that's all they may be helpful for.

IMPORTANT NOTE – if you are currently taking this type of medication, please be fully aware of its addictive nature and of the risks involved if you suddenly stop taking it. Instead, if you want to remove it from your life, gradual withdrawal under the guidance and monitoring of a medical professional is essential.

The other option offered is some sort of talking therapy or Cognitive Behavioural Therapy (CBT). I've spoken to people who say this has helped them a lot. But if I then ask if they're now well, the answer tends to be a sheepish look followed by something like, 'not really, but I'm getting there.' This has sometimes been after a year or more of such therapy.

As with the medication approach, the autonomic nervous system imbalance isn't caused by a lack of conversation with a stranger well trained in fixed ideas. However, as mentioned earlier, I do think that talking with a sympathetic, trusted friend or family member can be constructive and liberating. To be fair, though, perhaps some talking therapies might be helpful to an extent in certain circumstances, and they are, in my opinion, a better solution than medication, though not as readily available.

So, what then?

Dealing with stress

There are many things you can do to relieve stress, such as deep diaphragmatic breathing, mindfulness practice, which I look at in another chapter, listening to relaxing music, taking regular relaxation breaks throughout the day etc, and these things can be very beneficial. But please note that I said 'relieve', and they do, but I don't think they get to the crux of the matter when dealing with chronic stress.

If I was to ask you what's causing you to be stressed, what would your answer be? My boss drives me crazy? I'm stuck in traffic two hours a day just getting to work? My partner is seeing someone else? The kids drive me round the bend? There are hundreds of possibilities, often several going on at the same time. But they're not reasons, they're excuses. The fact is that there's only one cause of the stress you're experiencing, and that cause is YOU. What! Sorry, but it's true.

A stressor, any stressor, can't harm you in any way, but your reaction to that stressor can, big time. For example, imagine the two drivers in the traffic jam that I've just mentioned. One, with furrowed brow is angrily gripping the steering wheel, sounding his horn at every opportunity, gritting his teeth and cursing the time being wasted. The other is philosophical about the situation, putting his travel time to good use by listening to educational CDs or calming music. He has a smile on his face. They're both being subjected to the exact same stressor, but which one do you think is most likely to have a heart attack as some point?

Whatever the stressor is, you have three options.

1) Get stressed and damage your health, perhaps seriously.

2) Avoid the stressor, though this isn't always practicable–If you rely on the boss who drives you crazy and you have a mortgage, and there's no other job available, for example. But if it is reasonably easy to avoid, avoid it. This isn't the whole answer because you're controlling the situation rather than correcting your attitude towards it, but at least it lessens the load in the short to medium term.

3) Change your attitude towards the stressor. If your partner is seeing someone else, for example, talk to them, express your sadness and calmly ask 'why', then listen. Maybe you can resolve the situation, and if you can, reject any bitterness you might feel and forgive your partner and yourself for your joint failings. That forgiveness is very important. Then forget the past and look only forward. You have a new beginning, so grasp it. But maybe a resolution can't be found, in which case, be philosophical. With no hard feelings, separate and move on.

Whatever the situation, changing your attitude to what's stressing you is always possible, there's always a way. Sometimes that way is difficult to accept, and you may have to give something up. But if you continue to live in 'fight or flight' mode, you'll most likely develop anxiety or worse. You'll never be happy and content, and being happy and content is key to a good, healthy, worthwhile long life.

I've mentioned this in another chapter, but I feel it's important enough to bear repeating, I'd strongly suggest that you stop watching, listening to or reading the news. Why? Because the media doesn't give you, 'Young girl plays happily with her pet dog, and they love each other.' Instead, it gives you, 'Young girl savaged by pet dog'. They know that bad news is what sells their product, so that's what they give you, and what they give you is stress creating. You might not notice the stress at the time, but your subconscious will, and your subconscious takes programme building notes. But I need to know what's going on in the world, you might say. Why? What personal benefit have you ever gained by 'knowing what's going on in the world'?

Also, I'd suggest that you stop watching violent movies or the 'realistic' type of TV series that is so prevalent these days. They're stressful. Watch 'You've Been Framed' or something similar instead. Or read a funny book. Laugh, or at least smile. Both are great ways to evaporate stress.

Dealing with anxiety and panic attacks.

Chronic anxiety and panic attacks are due to your

subconscious creating powerful feelings of fear in you when there's no actual danger to justify that fear. I think it's very important to understand that. I suspect that sometime in your past you were subject to something so powerfully negative that your subconscious instantly wrote a programme designed to protect you from that something in the future, perhaps by creating the physical symptoms of anxiety as a warning should it happen or shows signs of happening again.

Unfortunately, your subconscious may create those same symptoms when anything it considers similar, however loosely, to that earlier experience. So even the slightest stressor can set you off. The solution is to overwrite that programme, though when dealing with anxiety and panic attacks, doing so requires courage.

I'm sorry, but you have to habitually face your demons until a new, positive programme is in place. If I knew of an easier way, I'd tell you, but every other option I've read about doesn't work, or only works temporarily or can easily be retriggered if some new stressful situation arises in your life. And, of course, such situations will arise in your life, probably on a regular basis.

The key point that should be kept at the forefront of your mind is that all you are facing is fear, but not just fear, fear of the fear that may well have been implanted many years previously. I fully appreciate that facing that fear can initially create even more fear, but that's why courage is a requirement.

So, if there is something specific that you know creates fear in you, perhaps leaving the house, for example, do it anyway, preferably with a trusted friend or family member being there to support and reassure you, especially when you first set off on this journey. If at first you can only make it to the front door, that's fine, but keep making that trip to the door until you realise and accept that nothing terrible is going to happen to you when you do. Reaching that point represents real progress, so pat yourself on the back.

Then, go to the front gate, then to the end of the street, then to the nearest shop, then beyond, each in turn as many times as it takes to achieve the same realisation and acceptance that you achieved at the front door. Baby steps are fine, but it's important to congratulate yourself for each success. Eventually, the old programme will be overwritten and your fear will be gone.

However long this process takes is how long it takes. For some, positive results will happen quite quickly, but for others, progress will be slower. That doesn't matter, because if you persist it WILL happen eventually, and even if it takes six months, isn't it better to sacrifice those six months than to spend a lifetime in fear of the front door?

But sometimes, although your subconscious knows what created your current episode, you may not. When this is the case, you need a distraction. But first, please be fully aware that you've been here before, and although you felt terrible, nothing bad happened and the anxiety faded. Say to yourself, repeatedly if necessary, 'well nothing bad happened before, so nothing bad is going to happen this time. This anxiety will soon pass as it has always done.' Then go and do something to distract your mind from it. Have a shower, splash lots of cold water on your face, listen to music, vacuum a carpet, take the dog for a walk, anything, but just do it.

Panic attacks are a bit different in that although they're simply an extension or escalation of anxiety, they're a truly terrifying thing to experience, one that can create the belief that you're about to collapse and die at any moment.

If you're new to panic attacks, I'd strongly advise you to seek urgent medical advice in order to be reassured that there's nothing physically wrong going on, like a heart attack, for example. But once it has been medically confirmed that your symptoms were caused by a panic attack, you must accept the fact, that's absolutely essential. If you don't, if you convince yourself that the doctor missed something vital, even life threatening, whilst examining you, you'll never stop the attacks from happening, and you'll probably go through that terrible experience again and again, possibly for life.

As with anxiety, panic attacks stem from fear of fear but at an acute and much more intense level. But I think resolution is relatively simple if the courage is there, so be brave. Here's what I'd suggest –

1) bring to the forefront of your mind that it's happened before, perhaps many times, and that you didn't die.

2) don't give in to it by laying down.

3) Face it head-on, say something like, 'bring it on, do your worst, you can be defeated, I'm not your

victim, I'm taking control, so sod off!' Feel free to use a stronger expletive than I've used here, the stronger the better because that will reinforce the power of your statement. And most importantly, say it with as much confidence as you can muster. Believe it.

However bad you feel, and you will feel bad, hold that 'I'm not your victim' thought until things settle down. You may have to do this many, many, times, but after each time, you'll get a little stronger. It's a good idea to keep a record of how much easier it was than before to recover from each experience, then refer to your record regularly. Doing so will build confidence and accelerate your progress to wellness.

Having said that, whilst I really do believe that facing panic attacks head on is the way to eliminate them long term, I do appreciate that there may be times when they are overwhelming. At such times, a quick fix is to breath in and out of a paper bag that covers your nose and mouth until things calm down. This rebalances your oxygen/carbon dioxide ratio and is usually very effective. But I must stress that I'd do this only in acute, severe situations. It's not a long-term solution.

Finally, I'd like to mention that I was helped a lot by the writing of Claire Weekes, an Australian who was very prominent in this field during the nineteen-sixties. Her books and audios are available on Amazon.

CHAPTER TWENTY-FIVE

Mindfulness

'Do not dwell in the past, do not dream of the future, concentrate the mind on the present moment'
– Buddha

'If you want to conquer the anxiety of life, live in the moment, live in the breath.' **– Amit Ray**

I've come across people who suggest that to practice mindfulness you must be a Buddhist. That's nonsense. And I've come across people who suggest that hours and hours of daily practice are required to achieve proficiency. Not true. I've seen much complex instruction, and I once bought a two-hundred-and-fifty-page book talking of nothing else. I lost interest at about page sixty, and it went to a local charity shop where it may well still reside.

To my mind, mindfulness is a simple concept that with practice, and yes, its mastery does require some practice, can be hugely beneficial.

What benefits does it offer?

In the past, life was fairly simple, though not especially pleasant unless you were rich. For most people, aspirations were low and objectives were few, perhaps to have sufficient food, to have warm clothes and somewhere to live that kept the rain out. If you had those things, there wasn't too much going on in terms of stress.

Today though, we've become competitive, we're subject to images of things we want but can't afford. There's a pecking order and we want to be higher up that order. Shopping is far more complex than it was, and the supermarkets where we shop offer an overwhelming array of confusing options. From an early age, our school children are driven to compete with their fellow pupils to be top of the class, to win cups on sports day, to pass exams, to go to university. There are mortgages and car payments to support, and a holiday to fund. There's something that has to be done every minute of the day, and if we can't do it, we feel we've failed, at least at the subconscious level. Then there's the chronic use of things like smartphones and social media, a perceived need to constantly check for texts or to see who's looking at our last social media offering.

Or maybe we develop a serious chronic illness, and never having had the opportunity to build capital to fall back on, we have to rely on benefits that barely cover the basic necessities, never mind the mortgage payments. This can create debilitating feelings of worthlessness that, whilst being invalid, nonetheless seem real.

All of the above can overwhelm our senses, creating stress and anxiety that builds feelings of failure in the battle to compete. Our minds are full of darting thoughts, mostly negative, that never stop piling on the pressure.

Mindfulness practice is a way to escape these constant thought processes and everything else that can overwhelm us, and if only for a few minutes a day, such escape can be tremendously beneficial. I've heard it said that ten minutes of mindfulness practice is worth two hours of quality sleep.

So what's the process and how is the process executed?

Mindfulness is being focused on 'the now'. For the time that you're in a mindfulness state, all the pressures outlined above are relieved, providing total respite from them. It really is that simple. How the previously mentioned author managed to fill two hundred and fifty pages on the subject I'll never know.

The process

Trying to quieten then clear your mind, replacing what was there with one thing, whether that be a word, an object or whatever, isn't easy at first, and may provoke an 'oh blow it' response that puts you off trying again. That would be a shame because it really is worth persevering. To minimise the risk of this happening, perhaps start with just a minute or so of practice, free of over ambitious expectations.

To begin, find a quiet place to sit or lie down, though this won't be necessary when you've become proficient. Next, take four or five deep, slow diaphragmatic breaths of the sort that forces your belly out, then catch the attention of one thing within or around you. It could be your breathing, for example. If so, note and explore all the movements and sensations that the breathing creates, like those of your belly pushing against your clothing, the feel of the air entering via your nose and leaving via your mouth etc. When a stray thought enters your mind, don't fight it. Simply acknowledge it, let it go and return to your breathing. Stray thoughts don't represent failure, it's in our nature to invite them in and they're to be expected. Don't let them frustrate you. They're part of the process, and as long as you return to your practice each time you let one go, that's fine.

It doesn't have to be your breathing, it could be a mark on the wall, a positive word, an object within your line of sight, a thought, anything at all, as long as you can focus your mind on it, and absorb everything about it that your senses can tell you. Gradually and without putting pressure on yourself, build up to ten or fifteen minutes. It's that simple. Just practice, willingly accepting any sessions that don't work as you'd wish as being part of the learning process.

In short, the objective is to rest your mind from all the intrusive thoughts of the past or the future, the thoughts where all your worries and stressors reside, and to be in 'the moment' where there is no worry or stress. As you develop the ability to be in 'the moment', you'll feel a calmness that you probably haven't felt for a very long time. Your muscle tension will soften and your autonomic nervous system will switch from sympathetic, alert for danger, to parasympathetic, calm and relaxed, all without you realising it. It's a beautiful and immensely therapeutic feeling.

CHAPTER TWENTY-SIX

Visualisation And Affirmations

'To bring anything into your life, imagine that it's already there.' – **Richard Bach**

'Visualize this thing that you want. See it, feel it, believe in it. Make your mental blueprint, and begin to build.' – **Robert Collier**

'Affirmations are our mental vitamins, providing the supplementary positive thoughts we need to balance the barrage of negative events and thoughts we experience daily.' – **Tia Walker**

I honestly believe that visualisation and affirmations are a helpful way to connect to your subconscious, and that they do, therefore, warrant some serious attention.

The idea is quite simple, in that visualisation is seeing yourself in the situation that you want to be in, and affirmations are verbalisation of the visualisation to provide the visualisation with added strength.

The theory, and I think it's more than a theory, is that done often enough, your subconscious will take what you visualise as an instruction and make arrangements to set the achievement ball rolling by creating conscious thoughts that encourage any required action. For example, if part of your healing requires taking vitamin C, the thought of taking vitamin C might enter your consciousness.

When you're chronically ill, it's well worth giving some thought to what you think about and see in your mind's eye most of the time. It's likely that what you think about and see more or less constantly is yourself in a situation of poor health. If you can accept that your mind is at least influenced by your conscious thoughts, then this clearly can't be a good thing, and it must make sense to direct your thoughts to a better place on a regular basis.

The word visualisation implies clearly seeing in the conventional sense, as in the moving pictures on a TV screen. Often with practice and occasionally at the first attempt, some people can visualise like that, but many people can't, so they give up on the process, never gaining the benefit of a potentially useful tool.

But for visualisation to work effectively, it's certainly not essential to create pictures in your mind's eye. It's great if you can, but it's not necessary. You can visualise effectively by just 'feeling it', 'sensing it' or 'thinking about it'. In short, not everyone is visually oriented, but those who aren't can still benefit from this practice.

Once the process is underway, it's quite important that you're not too enthusiastic in terms of what you're going to achieve. I'm not sure that anyone has a perfect belief system that can achieve the seemingly impossible on its own, (maybe Jesus had such a belief system, though?), so in the short term, it's wise to aim for something that you see as being unlikely but possible.

So if you were once a marathons runner but have been

bed-bound for two years, initially, it makes sense to visualise yourself doing something like pottering around the house or perhaps doing a bit of dusting, or whatever, rather than visualising running your next marathon. When that pottering has been achieved, you'll gain confidence, which will in turn strengthen your belief system. So you can then choose a new goal to visualise. When that next goal has been achieved, you can move on to the next then the next and so on until, finally, it'll seem reasonable to visualise running that marathon. For most of us, steps of faith rather than leaps are the way forward.

One key issue is to see, sense, feel or think about what you're visualising as though it already exists. You may feel that that's just self-deceit, but it isn't. Everything you've ever seen, sensed, felt or thought about that came into existence did so because you believed that it would. Therefore, it did exist as a belief, and the energy of that belief alone brought it into being on the physical plane.

Regarding affirmations, I wrote about these in the 'Mind programmes and genetics' chapter but feel that a degree of reiteration is warranted here.

As mentioned earlier in this chapter, affirmations are used simply to strengthen the visualisation. So let's say you're comfortably visualising a pleasant walk on the beach on a warm sunny day. Then you might say to yourself something along the lines of, 'I'm enjoying this, it's very warm, but that sea breeze is really refreshing, the sand between my toes feels good, and I might go for a swim later.' Affirmations can be spoken aloud, but if like me you're uncomfortable with that, silently in your head is fine.

It's very important to visualise and affirm very regularly, and not get despondent if nothing seems to be happening in the short term. Like so many of the suggestions in this book, practice, time and patience are required. Also, initially, I'd suggest concentrating your efforts on one objective at a time, one you feel is achievable, then moving on to the next when it has been achieved.

Necessarily, the above is just a simple introduction to a concept that I'm sure from personal experience really does help you connect to your subconscious and create a better future. If you'd like something more in-depth, 'Creative Visualisation' by Shakti Gawain is a short but really good and instructive read.

Finally, I used to think this sort of thing was hogwash, and you might be thinking something similar now, but it has certainly helped me. So please try to maintain an open mind, because helpful options for chronic illness recovery are limited, and this one might just be the missing piece of your particular health building jigsaw.

PART FOUR

Emotional and Spiritual Considerations

Chapter 27 – Negative emotions

Chapter 28 – Positive emotions

Chapter 29 – Spirituality

CHAPTER TWENTY-SEVEN

Negative Emotions

'Spring is coming.... Time for some cleaning. Remove all the self-doubt, worry, jealousy, regret, anger, guilt, or any other negative emotions that are holding you back from your happy, fulfilled life.'
– **Nanette Mathews**

'Cultivate love within you and all your negative emotions will soon disappear.' – **Sri Avinash Do**

'Overthinking arises when you unconsciously provoke negative emotions and thoughts and avoid positive emotions and thoughts.' – **Amit Ray**

'Negative emotional states are a breeding ground for mistakes.' – **Sam Owen**

Make no mistake, negative emotions, especially the biggies like hate and resentment, can kill you. That's a fact.

When I set out to write this part of my book, I thought long and hard about how far I should go into this incredibly complex subject, eventually deciding that it is too big a subject to be covered in one chapter. So in the end I changed tack, deciding on a different and much simpler way forward.

I may well meander a bit here, but if I do, please bear

with me because I believe that what I'm going to talk about, which is by no means a quick fix, was one of the major keys to my health turnaround.

I'm rubbish at remembering when things happened, and initially, I'd have said this part of my story began about five years ago. But then I recalled that I bought the book that I'll come to shortly not long after it was published in the UK. I've just checked, and that was in June 2007. So this story actually began around twelve years ago, and although I was way out on my timing, I can remember quite clearly what happened to set the ball rolling.

I'd made a little progress towards recovery, but looking back, that progress was really quite limited. I wasn't bedbound then, but walking a few yards made me feel really ill, and recovery from the slightest physical exertion could take weeks. I went out for lunch occasionally and I clearly remember standing in a short queue at a carvery one day, convinced that I was about to die. I'd done everything that I could think of, but I couldn't get beyond this point and I was stuck where I didn't want to be. Looking back, I suspect that some degree of depression was involved, but whatever, I was in a dark place.

At that time, I subscribed to several health website newsletters, and I regularly received emails from them extolling the virtues of this, that or the other. One morning, I received one that recommended a book. For me, reading was very difficult back then, but not knowing why, I ordered the book. It arrived a few days later, and despite my difficulties, I read it quite quickly.

It seemed weird and farcical, talking of things related to emotions that just seemed daft–new age rubbish, basically. Disappointed, my mind closed to what the book was saying, I put it on a shelf where it remained for quite a few years.

During those years, amongst others, I read some of Einstein's and Bruce Lipton's work, getting to learn a bit about energy and how energy works, and that everything is energy and nothing is solid, and that energies we can't see influence the shape of physical structures via a vortex with protons bouncing off, creating the illusion of solidity. This is an area that seriously interests me but in which I have no deep knowledge. So if you're a quantum physicist, please forgive me for errors of explanation.

Then one day, again not knowing why, I picked the book up again and started to reread it. This time it resonated, perhaps influenced by the reading I'd been doing in the interim. The principles started to make sense to me and I began to put them into practice.

Slowly but surely, I became really intrigued, and as I became more proficient in using the techniques explained in the book, improvements in health began to materialise. I have no doubt whatsoever that, as I said at the beginning of this chapter, this was a major key to my health turnaround.

It took around a year before that turnaround became seriously meaningful, but were it not for this book, I'm quite sure that I'd still be where I was, or close to where I was, at the beginning of my journey.

So why am I telling you all this? Well when I set out to write this chapter, attempting to set out the principles and practices I'd learned, it eventually occurred to me that it made far more sense to just suggest that you read the book.

It's titled **'The Emotion Code'.by Dr Bradley Nelson.**

I can't of course guarantee that it will be as much value to you as it was to me, but I really do think it's worth considering, as long as you treat it as a study book rather than as a quick read that will solve all your emotional issues overnight. It won't, and you'll regret the purchase as I did on first reading.

You might say that you don't have any emotional issues, and perhaps you'd be right. But I'd venture to suggest that you're probably wrong. As someone with a chronic disease, don't you ever worry, are you ever fearful of the future, do you ever long for your old life, do you ever feel overwhelmed, do you feel vulnerable, or helpless, or frustrated, or anxious, or unsupported, or worthless, or sad, or even a little bit bitter? These and many others are all negative emotions, and negative emotions can seriously hurt you physically.

Furthermore, it's extremely likely that you have emotions that are so strong and destructive that your subconscious mind has, in an attempt to protect you, removed them from your conscious memory, storing their energy in the tissues of your physical body where they can be incredibly destructive.

And emotions can be inherited going back as far as fourteen generations, so you might even be suffering from an emotion that was created in someone else several centuries ago. The Emotion Codes author, Dr Bradley Nelson, knew this years ago, but recent epigenetic research has confirmed it.

But what matters is that all these 'trapped' emotions can be released. The book explains all this and much more, and as long as you have a truly open mind, and assuming you're not expecting that a quick read will solve all your problems, I really do believe it has the potential to be of tremendous long-term value to you.

There are many alternative energy healing modalities, and I've looked into most of them and tried a few. I can honestly say that 'The Emotion Code' is the one that has seriously impressed and helped me.

An initial alternative to buying the book is to Google 'emotion code gift', scroll down to 'The Emotion Code – video series" and click.

Finally, if anyone is interested in the concept but prefers the practitioner approach, there are now many practitioners scattered around the world, and if there isn't one near you, I understand that some of them can consult by phone or Skype. Just Google 'emotion code practitioners'

CHAPTER TWENTY-EIGHT

Positive Emotions

'We all live at the mercy of our emotions. Our emotions influence and shape our desires, thoughts and behaviours and above all our destiny' – **Dr T P Chia**

'The way to overcome negative thoughts and destructive emotions is to develop opposing, positive emotions that are stronger and more powerful.' – **Dalai Lama**

'Positive and negative emotions cannot occupy the mind at the same time. One or the other must dominate. It is your responsibility to make sure that positive emotions constitute the dominating influence of your mind. Here emotions" will come to your aid. Form the habit of applying and using the positive emotions! Eventually, they will dominate your mind so completely, that the negatives cannot enter it.' – **Napoleon Hill**

When you've started to release negative emotions, it's a very good idea to begin creating positive ones, ones that release chemicals that make you happy and keep you happy and, perhaps more importantly, reduce stress, thus improving your digestive process, enhancing your immune system's function and, above all, encouraging improved health and wellbeing.

A good starting point is learning to be calm and relaxed as best you can. Reflect on the good things in your life and, again as best you can, reduce your exposure to the hamster wheel that is a major element of modern life. Perhaps give up some of your TV time and give it over to meditation, or listening to calming music, or anything else that you find calming. Stop or at least severely limit watching, reading or listening to the news, which ninety-nine percent of the time has no bearing on you or your life and is renowned for its negativity.

These things will reduce your attention to the things that create negative emotions and increase it to the things that create positive ones, and you may well be pleasantly surprised by how much better your life becomes. I know there are limits to how much you can slow your life down, and that we can't all live in a quiet little village full of calm, happy people relaxing around the duck pond, but do the best you can. Any reduction in exposure to modern madness will help.

There are numerous positive emotions, but to my mind there are four that are more important than the rest and which encourage the rest to come into being. Those four are forgiveness, gratitude, charity and love. I've discussed forgiveness elsewhere in this book, so here, I'd like to touch on the other three.

Gratitude

If you have a chronic illness, you can be forgiven for thinking that you have nothing to be grateful for, but if you consider for a while, I'm sure you'll find at least a few. In fact, I'd like you to do your best to come up with ten. Things like your children, your partner, your grandchildren, your dog or cat, the fact that you have a roof over your head etc.

How will doing this help you? If you spend a few moments each day contemplating your list, what's on it will replace, or a least reduce, the things in your mind that you're not grateful for. And if you do this regularly, those things will become less and less troublesome. Please give it a try, and don't give up too soon.

Charity

Some might say that charity isn't an emotion, but I disagree. Charitable thoughts are positive thoughts, and positive thoughts create positive emotions. I know that chronically ill people tend to have limited financial means, but charity isn't just about giving money to good causes. It's also about giving someone in trouble a helping hand or a shoulder to cry on, or a kind, supportive word. Basically, it can refer to anything that involves the word 'give', and giving certainly isn't just about material gifts. In fact, the non-material gifts are often those most valued by their recipient.

Of course giving to good causes is a positive thing, but if doing so is unaffordable, there is an option that I've been doing every morning for at least ten years via a website called www.thehungersite.com. If you log on to this site and click on 'click to give' you've provided a bowl of rice to someone living in a third world country and who is in dire need. That may not seem much, but if just one percent of the UK population did this every day, that would provide a great deal of free rice for those who are desperate for it. And it takes less than two minutes to do.

How will doing these things help you? It's often said that 'it's better to give than to receive', and that's true. Helping someone else helps you too, because, trust me, you'll feel better and more worthwhile than you do now.

Love

To my mind, love is the king of positive emotions. If you have religious affinities, you'll read of its importance throughout your scriptures. When John Lennon told us that 'all you need is love', I was tempted to argue a point. After all, we need a sandwich every now and then, but conceptually, I agree with him one-hundred percent. The direct opposite of love is hate, and the reason they're opposites is that loving attracts love whereas hating is like taking poison expecting the person you hate to die. So in emphasis, it's far more destructive to you, the hater, than it is to the subject of your hate. But when you love someone, it's great for them, but it's even greater for you, because love attracts love, and love is the greatest non-medicinal healer of all.

So I'd suggest to everyone that you love all living things – plants, animals and people. When you eat plants and animals, love them for providing you with life by giving their lives. That can be difficult if you're eating factory farmed animals that have had no real life, but if you eat pastured and well cared for animals, the good life they've given up is a life they wouldn't otherwise have had.

Finally, you don't have to like someone to love them. All you have to do is accept them as they are and understand that you have no idea what happened in their past that made them what they are – there but for the grace of God go I. Wish them well regardless of their character. That's what love is, and it benefits you tremendously.

As I suggested earlier, these three positive emotions along with forgiveness are the seeds from which other positive emotions have the potential to grow, so sow and nurture them as best you can. You can only benefit by doing so.

CHAPTER TWENTY-NINE

Spirituality

'Everything is energy, and the material field is simply a reflection of the invisible field **(Spirit?)** *– Quantum Physics'* – **brackets mine.**

'Ask and it will be given to you; seek and you will find; knock and the door will be opened to you. For everyone who asks receives; the one who seeks finds; and to the one who knocks, the door will be opened' – **Matthew 7:7-8**

Before I start this chapter, I'm very aware that you may have no interest in spirituality, and in my world that's fine. It took me over sixty-five years to introduce myself to it and embrace it as being part of the whole me – physical, mental, emotional and spiritual. You might at some point find a connection or you may not. But whether you do or whether you don't is also fine with me. We must each find our own way through life.

But for those who do have a belief, there are many roads to spirituality and it's right that we should all choose our own.

I subscribe to the first quote above. I believe that 'the invisible field', which I'll refer to as Spirit, is all powerful and can influence our lives tremendously in positive ways if we invite it to do so.

Because we have free will though, we have to ask for guidance. I'm not going into great detail, but Spirit first came into my life during a time when I was at a loss regarding what to do next. I actually asked for help with no idea who I was asking, but shortly afterwards, all sorts of useful information came into my consciousness from all manner of physical resources. I'm slightly ashamed to admit that it was some time before I joined the dots and connected my request to what followed, but I now connect on a daily basis, and that connection has been immensely beneficial.

Personally, I have absolutely no religious affiliations, but if you do have, then I'd ask you to consider the second quote above. Whichever religion you subscribe to, I'm sure you'll recognise what's written there, or there'll be very similar words in your particular scriptures. Yes, you recognise them, but have you really considered then acted on them? If so, then you don't need to read further. But if not, I believe my Spirit guide to be incredibly powerful, but because of the teachings you've received, and the beliefs that you've developed from those teachings, your God will be equally powerful, or for all I know, more so.

So, I'm not asking you to adopt my belief, but to take advantage of your own, and make contact with your God by expressing gratitude for what you do have and asking for a guidance path towards acquiring what you want but don't have. In the context of this book, that would be good health and wellbeing.

Based purely on my own experience, before you can make a sustainable connection to Spirit there needs to be sincerity in your request along with a deep need of some sort. Having made the request, please don't miss the connection between messages that follow and their source, like I did. Neither your God nor my Spirit shout out or create lightning flashes to catch your attention. Rather, what comes tends to be subtle to the extent that it's easily missed, and it's a great shame to miss it because it's invariably invaluable.

When I need an answer to something that I can't work out for myself, I use a simple muscle testing technique that I learned from 'The Emotion Code' book that I referred to in the positive emotions chapter. I also use a gesture that I've found reference to in many places that discuss these things. I understand that in certain quarters this gesture is a symbol of love. Whether it's necessary or even effective in any way, I'm not sure, but many people who walk a spiritual path with convictions deeper than mine believe it is. I really don't know, but I decided that they're more knowledgeable than I am in these matters, so I adopted it and it has now become a habit. The gesture is simply to fold the second and third fingers of your non-dominant hand into your palm then place your hand over your heart.

Perhaps there will be some readers who would like to know more about the technique I use, so I'll do my best to explain it below. But first, when I say 'simple muscle testing', I'm not talking about the practice of kinesiology, which takes years of practice to become proficient in, but about something very much simpler.

Step one–In as relaxed a state as possible, stand with your legs at shoulder width, and put in place the previously mentioned gesture. I don't know whether or not that's really necessary, but it's what I do.

Step two—Take a few moments to calm your mind, then physically ask for guidance followed by thanks for the guidance you'll receive. You may feel your body sway very slightly forward when you've done that. If so, that implies a strong connection. However, this is rare when trying for the first time, so don't be concerned if it doesn't happen.

Step three—Fill your mind with something really positive, perhaps a picture of your grandchild or a favourite pet. Anything that, to you, represents love. Then calmly wait. Don't want or expect anything to happen, that's important. Within a few seconds, your body may sway slightly forward. Now, think of something that, to you, represents something bad, evil even, but anything that really repulses you. Again within a few seconds, your body may sway slightly backwards. If this is what happens, the belief is that you've connected to your guide.

Step four. Assuming you did sway in step three, now say something you know to be true, your name, for example, in which case you'd say 'my name is whatever' you should sway slightly forward. Now say something you know to be false. Using the same thing, you could say, 'my name is—but lie'. You should sway slightly backwards.

Step five—If this experience has been successful, you can then start asking questions for guidance, questions that require only a yes or no answer, again, that's important. If yes, you'll sway forward, if no, you'll sway backwards. The more powerful the sway, the more important the answer. Don't do this for too long, though, because, initially, it is tiring. I'd suggest no more than five minutes. And ensure that you're well hydrated. For some reason, this is necessary.

If the experience has failed, drink a glass of water and try again. If it still fails, maintain an open mind and try several times over the next few days. If you still have no success, then perhaps the more in-depth explanation in the previously mentioned book might help, or perhaps this practice just isn't for you, and hopefully, you'll find something that suits your purpose better elsewhere.

However, if this practice has worked for you, it can be extremely useful in the future. When I started to do it, I kept records for several weeks then reviewed these records. The answers to questions that I couldn't find my own answers to, proved to be ninety-seven percent accurate. I suspect that the three percent failures were either due to dehydration or me being in the wrong frame of mind at the time.

So, a spiritual connection? A simple connection to the subconscious? The high hit rate just being down to coincidence? I really don't know, though I suspect the former. Whatever, this practice has been of immense value to me.

I have found that this helps when asking questions personal to me, but it isn't designed to help you win the lottery or whatever. In fact, I'd suggest that to attempt things like that would be an abuse of the practice.

A thought that's just occurred to me is that perhaps my spiritual guide was mainly responsible for this book. In fact, it's quite possible that I was only employed to do the typing. Yes, my tongue is in my cheek, but you never know.

Finally, to reiterate what I said at the start of the chapter, if you have no interest in spirituality, that's absolutely fine. It took me many decades to find mine. And if you never find that interest, that's fine, too. What really matters is, and I unashamedly quote from the Christian bible, that you 'do unto others as you would have them do unto you' (Luke 6:31).

PART FIVE

In Closing

Chapter 30 – Snippets

Conclusion

……And finally

References

Glossary

Fiction by Roger Knowles

CHAPTER THIRTY

Snippets

This final chapter consists of snippets that didn't find a chapter of their own but which I feel are nonetheless worthy of inclusion in this book.

Sleep

Adequate sleep is essential, and I don't believe that good health is achievable without it. But how much sleep do we need? Some 'experts' will insist that if you don't get seven to eight hours every night your head will explode or your leg will fall off. Well I've gone to bed more than twenty-six-thousand times, and I don't remember ever getting more than six hours, more often five. My head and legs are still safely intact. We're all different and our needs vary, and I think what really matters is how you feel when you wake up. If you're refreshed and ready for the new day, then I'd suggest that you'll be fine. But what if you wake up not feeling refreshed and ready for the new day?

You'll find all the standard advice all over the internet, so I won't go into that here, but I do have a few thoughts. Sleep is governed by hormones. Melatonin puts you to sleep and serotonin and GABA, when properly balanced with glutamate in the brain, keeps you asleep. So, if you have trouble getting to sleep, maybe try a melatonin supplement, and if you wake up when you shouldn't, maybe try serotonin, or its precursor 5-HTP, valerian root or PharmaGABA – please note that you'll find GABA everywhere but in my experience it doesn't work terribly well. You need PharmaGABA. However, before trying these things, I'd suggest first try a good quality lavender essential oil, either by adding a few drops to your pillow, or breathing it from the bottle or from an essential oil inhaler. It's amazing how often this works.

Having said all that, I find that, given time, a simple affirmation can work well. Every night without fail, just before sleep, whether I need to or not, I say, *'tonight I'll get the right sleep in terms of length, depth and quality to ensure all aspects of my being receive the rest, relaxation and rejuvenation they need to ensure continuing good health and wellbeing.'* That's my approach but anything similar in your own words would be fine. This approach is unlikely to work well immediately, but if you persist, your subconscious mind should eventually get the message and act accordingly.

Finally, I think the worst thing you can do if you can't get to sleep or if you wake up in the early hours is to worry about it, because that creates stress hormones and these as extremely good at eliminating all hope of a good night's sleep. So, my advice would be don't concern yourself. Just be philosophical about it and accept the situation. Relax as best you can and think nice thoughts, perhaps contemplating ten things that you're grateful for. That can be very calming.

Purpose

For life to be really worthwhile, it needs a meaningful purpose, and having such a purpose is an incredibly powerful healer, physically, mentally and emotionally. Of course, throughout life there will be many purposes – things you want to achieve – and you'll succeed in some and fail in others, the failures being valuable because they're educational.

In the context of this book, the purpose is to correct imbalances and achieve good health and wellbeing, it being about how I did that, and I hope it has provided some useful ideas for you. But at the end of the day, whether or not you get well depends on finding an approach that works for you whether from here or elsewhere. Whatever, wishing and hoping won't help you do that, but in my experience, belief and commitment will. Have a plan and execute it. And when you've recovered your health, it'll be time to find a new purpose, because continually having a positive purpose is what life is or should be about.

Infections

The only things I have in my emergency medicine cabinet are colloidal silver, oregano oil, vitamin C and hydrogen peroxide. They've never let me down.

Salt

Salt is heavily demonised, and in the case of table salt and salt in processed food, that demonization is justified. But we do need salt. To replace the bad stuff, try Himalayan salt, which has sodium but lots of other micro minerals too. Celtic sea salt is also good, as long as it's grey, not white. But it's no good for sprinkling on food, whereas fine ground Himalayan salt is.

Eggs

There are still 'experts' saying that the cholesterol in eggs will give us heart disease. It won't. They also tell us that the saturated fat in eggs will clog our arteries. It won't. The reality is that eggs contain vitamins A, B, D, E and K. Additionally, they contain the minerals selenium, calcium, zinc and phosphorus, and one egg gives you about six grams of good quality protein. They also contain the antioxidants lutein and zeaxanthin. Additionally, eggs from pastured chickens provide essential omega 3 fatty acids. If ever a single food could be described as super nutritious, that food would be eggs, ideally organic but at least free range pastured.

Sex

Yes, I know you probably feel rubbish and that the notion of sex doesn't excite you at the moment, but it doesn't have to be the swinging from the chandeliers type. It can be gentle and sensual and it has many health benefits. For example – it boosts the immune system, it reduces stress, it gets more blood to the brain thus increasing brainpower, even gentle sex is good exercise, it releases lots of good hormones including those that reduce pain, it improves sleep, it keeps you younger than you'd be without it – the list goes on. If you have a partner who understands your condition, maybe suggest getting back into the groove, but stress the need for a slow and gentle approach, perhaps preceded by a shared bath or a sensual massage If you don't have a partner, whatever the vicar told you, there's no shame in self sex, which still has many of the aforementioned benefits as long as there's no unjustified guilt involved.

Bad thought and memories

Your thoughts and memories are the government of a community, that community being your many trillions of cells. If these thoughts and memories are positive, this community is in growth mode, where everything is working as it was designed to do. But if your thoughts and memories are negative, the community goes into protection mode where nothing much is being done, resulting in a state of stagnation, which is a very unhealthy state.

We've all done bad things in the past and we've all had bad things done to us. But where's the benefit in hanging on to the thoughts and memories of such things? There is no benefit. Forgive everyone involved, including yourself, and let the memories go. As for bad thoughts, change them, as discussed elsewhere in this book.

Microwave cooking

The research on microwave cooking is mixed – some very pro and some very anti and some undecided. On balance, I decided against using a microwave oven some years ago on the basis that as microwaves, from mobile phones, for example, are harmful to me, they're probably harmful and denaturing to what I eat. Since then, I've never come across research that would make me change my mind.

Breathing

When you have a chronic illness, there's a tendency for your autonomic nervous system to be out of whack, making you sympathetic (fight or flight) dominant. When this is the case, there's a further tendency to develop over breathing (breathing too fast) or erratic breathing, which sometimes develops into unconscious breath holding. This isn't good because it disrupts your oxygen/CO2 balance, which in turn results in less oxygen getting to your cells.

At rest, you should be breathing no more than twelve times a minute and preferably less than that. So each in/out breath should take five seconds or longer, and I think it's well worth checking your breathing rate. However, doing this yourself may give a false result because you'll probably consciously or subconsciously try to adjust in order to meet a target. Therefore, it's best to ask someone else to check your resting breathing rate when you don't know they're doing it.

If you find that your breathing is out of whack, meaning too quick, erratic or stopping every now and then, you can correct this overtime with deep belly breathing exercises that really push your belly out. You'll find various such exercises online, but I find that a count of five in and a count of seven out with a one second gap between works well. Beware though, that it does take some time to create a good breathing habit, so don't give up too soon.

You never know

Looking back, I think that getting the severe imbalances

that lived with me for so long was one of the best things that ever happened to me because I like who I am far more than I did previously, and I think I've grown as a person. It forced me to travel along a huge learning curve, and that journey has benefitted me tremendously in several ways. I'm telling you this because I'd like to ask you a favour. Next time you're experiencing a real low and you're having thoughts like, 'Why is this happening to me' or 'Why should I have to deal with this?' or just 'Why me?' try changing those thoughts to 'You never know', because you really don't. Maybe you're on a journey with a worthwhile destination, and maybe your current situation is a necessary part of that journey.

Exercise

Exercise is important, and if you are able to exercise with your particular chronic illness, that's good, though I'd advise against strenuous exercise of the type that creates lots of free radicals because creating more free radicals than necessary isn't a good idea when your body's trying to heal. But walking is fine. However, you may feel so ill that even walking isn't viable, as was the case with me for several years. If that's so in your case, don't fret about it. As things start to improve, you can then start a gentle walking programme.

But with or without the thoughts and ideas expressed in this book, my hope is that you'll find your way to wellness, and when you do, you'll need to think about regaining the physical fitness you lost while ill.

My suggestion for achieving that is rebounding. Why?

Because it's an exercise that works in so many ways and can be started very gently via what's called 'the health bounce', where you just stand on the rebounder bouncing slowly without your feet leaving the surface. That alone gets your lymph system working again, which is necessary for elimination of toxins. From there, you can gradually build intensity right up to a complete workout. In short, you can achieve a high level of fitness without risking harm, all from one simple activity.

When the time for this arrives, rebounders are available all over the internet. Get the best you can afford or perhaps consider a good quality used one, which again can be found online.

You can't dry off until you've left the shower

What do I mean by that? Whether you acquire useful information from this book or from elsewhere, health improvements will materialise, and that's good. But I think it's important to understand that to get and remain fully recovered you have to 'get out of the shower'. In other words, you have to deal with the underlying reason that caused you to become ill in the first place – if you're wet, and want to be dry, you have to remove yourself from the source of your wetness before you reach for a towel. If you don't, even though you may think you're recovering or have even recovered, if the circumstances that created your illness in the first-place still exist, that illness, (or some other one,) is likely to return at some point. The two most likely culprits that might return you to illness are, as I've suggested before, toxicity and deficiency, and this toxicity and/or deficiency can be physical, mental, emotional or spiritual.

So, if you feel you're getting well or indeed are well, complacency can be dangerous. It's a good idea to maintain the corrections you made during your journey, and to carefully examine your history to see if you can pinpoint any longstanding problem then deal with it once and for all.

Oral infections

Do you notice any blood when you clean your teeth? Do you have any amalgam fillings? Have you had an extraction when the dentist pulled the tooth and just left it at that? Do you have one or more root canals? Do you have any dental pain or 'strange' sensations?

If the answer to any of the above is 'yes', then you could have an unrecognised infection that is the root cause of your symptoms. In fact, it's well documented that such infections can spread throughout the body causing anything from heart disease, to diabetes to arthritis and to many other recognised chronic 'diseases'

This isn't the place to go into great detail, but if you answered 'yes' to any of those questions, my advice would be to get thoroughly checked out by a well-established holistic dentist, asking him to check you for an infected cavitation and to check any root canals–which are a major source of unrecognised whole body infections–and amalgam fillings, which contain mercury, a major neurotoxin.

Assumptions

> *Pussy cat, pussy cat where have you been*
> *Have you been to London to visit the queen?*
> *Where's London, what queen, said puss on my lap*
> *I've been in the greenhouse having a nap*

That's a light-hearted example of a ridiculous assumption proven wrong by a simple explanation. During my journey I assumed many things that proved to be wrong and would have been corrected by asking questions or doing a little research. Once an assumption has been made, it can appear to you as a reality, and accepting that 'reality' could delay your recovery, perhaps by years. So avoid assumptions, they'll lead you astray. Research and ask questions until you have a fact.

Keeping colds and flu at bay

My daily three grams of vitamin C certainly helps – see the supplement chapter – but what I believe really keeps me free of viral infections amongst other things are Zane Hellas Immune Premium total immune support soft gels, which contains extra virgin olive oil as a base, oregano essential oil, echinacea oil, ginseng oil, garlic oil, chios mastic oil, turmeric oil, ginger oil, and St John's wort oil – please note, if you have an autoimmune condition, ask your doctor before taking St John's wort, though the amount in the above combination is very small. Working in concert, these ingredients provide powerful immune support, intestinal support and digestive function support. I love them. They can sometimes be hard to find, but if

that's the case you'll find them at www.zanehellas.com
. They ship pretty much all over the world.

Hypnosis

Hypnosis can be briefly defined as an altered state of consciousness via trance, in which the hypnotised individual becomes more susceptible to positive and potentially health-giving suggestion than in his normal state.

During my search for answers, I got interested in hypnosis. I did my research and found an extremely well qualified clinical hypnotherapist who was a senior member of a prestigious association. His practice was less than ten miles from where I live. I phoned him and he assured me that he'd had a great deal of success with chronically ill people. His rate was one hundred and twenty pounds per session and the session would last between sixty and ninety minutes. He felt that four or five sessions would be required. That seemed a bit expensive, but, hey, he was a top man.

The day came and the hypnotherapist explained the procedure. During the session. I felt slightly uneasy without knowing why. About thirty minutes in, he told me I was in trance and that my symptoms were evaporating, though I knew I wasn't and that they weren't. In fact, they were getting worse. At forty-five minutes in, I felt extremely unwell, and I ended the session abruptly. I paid him and left.

I've been fixated on self-reliance and being in control of my own destiny since my early teens, and I believe that my inability to get on with hypnosis was due to an unwillingness to pass control to someone else. I know that's not a good trait, but it's one I'm stuck with.

I'm telling you this because I strongly suspect that the problem was mine rather than the hypnotherapist's, and I know of several people who've had great success via this route.

My point is that despite my own experience, I feel the subject of hypnosis has enough potential to at least be mentioned in this book. But as I have little knowledge to pass on, I felt I couldn't make a chapter of it. So, it's here as a snippet, as a reminder of its existence, because although it wasn't useful for me, it might be for you, and you might want to investigate its potential for your particular health issue.

Far Infrared saunas

I had a problem with sweating, in that I couldn't do it. I understood the importance of detoxifying, and that sweating was the number one way of doing that by washing out toxins through the skin. So I did some research and kept coming across the benefits of far infrared saunas, which come in many forms ranging in price from around three hundred pounds to over five thousand pounds. Having looked at the many options, I contacted a company called get-fitt.com, and spoke at length to the owner, Mark Givert. He recommended a far infrared sauna mat and I accepted the recommendation, with a thirty-day return promise if it proved unhelpful.

I almost returned it immediately because in less than

two minutes of use at the lowest temperature setting, I felt dreadful. I phoned to arrange the return and, again, had a long conversation with Mark regarding my particular health issues. When I mentioned severe mitochondrial disfunction, he knew what the problem was immediately. Far infrared has a mild exercise effect, and my body was unable to cope with that. He'd heard of this issue many times before and he suggested a protocol that would deal with it. It did, and after quite a few weeks, my ability to sweat gradually began to return. I now use my mat to good effect for around twenty minutes three to four times a week. So if you have an inability to sweat, it could be worth your while to investigate far infrared sauna therapy.

I bought mine from–www.get-fitt.com

Incidentally, research indicates the far infrared benefits go far beyond solving sweating problems. There is evidence that it can help patients with heart failure, COPD, arterial disease and several types of chronic pain, amongst other things.

Energy healing

There are many types of energy healing, and if the practitioner knows their craft, results can be amazing. Sadly, there are many practitioners who don't know their craft, and there are some outright fakes out there.

Luckily, I found one who does know her craft and has helped many, many people on their healing journey. She's a highly skilled kinesiologist, but over the years she's also developed many of her own highly effective energy healing skills that complement the kinesiology. She also trains others in the field of energy healing. Her name is Jay Cubitt and she got me over a hump – thank you, Jay. Her website is www.spectrum-healing.co.uk and she can do distance healing.

In Closing

'THE MOST IMPORTANT THING IN ILLNESS IS TO KEEP KISSING FROGS AND TO NEVER GIVE UP'–RK

This book began with my 'what I believe were the keys to my recovery' list, which I repeat below –

1. **Your diagnosis is just a label, and being wedded to it can hold you back.**

2. **Take responsibility. You're in charge. You. Nobody else.**

3. **There are four elements to you – physical, mental, emotional and spiritual. They must all be nurtured.**

4. **What you put in and, on your body becomes you – junk in, junk out.**

5. **Doctors aren't God – what they know is what they've been taught and not all of what they've been taught is true.**

6. **Digestion – achieving a well working digestive system is vital. All other physical elements are dependent on that.**

7. **Water – clean drinking water and lots of it, is extremely important.**

8. **Supplements. If you take supplements, quality**

really does matter, so don't skimp on price. If skimping on price is your only option, don't buy supplements.

9. **The two key causes of chronic illness are toxicity and deficiency, either physical, mental, emotional or spiritual, or any combination of these.**

It then went on to say that it was a list, lacking in detail, with much need for expansion and clarification, and that I'd attempt to provide that expansion and clarification in the following pages. I have strived to achieve that objective in the preceding chapters, and I hope I've succeeded. If you've found some information within my book's pages that has brought you relief in some way, I'll be very pleased. But if it has encouraged you to start on a fully-fledged healing journey, I'll be absolutely delighted. But if it has, accept that there may be disappointments along the way. If so, please don't give up, a mistake I nearly made several times. Rather, understand that the road will almost certainly have potholes, but that doesn't mean it can't be navigated. You never know what's around the next bend. An army of suitable frogs, perhaps?

Finally, I really do appreciate the fact that you've taken the time to read my book, and if you have any comments, whether positive or not, I'll be delighted to hear from you. I can be contacted at cargerbooks@gmail.com. I do receive many emails, so my response may be a little slow in coming, and I hope you'll forgive me for that, but it will come.

Roger Knowles 2019.

...And Finally

I've added this final section because I am very aware that some, perhaps many, who come across this book will condemn it on the basis of preaching quackery, at least in part. I understand and accept that opinion because it would also have been my opinion prior to beginning my healing journey.

However, I believe very strongly in the validity of what's written below and would ask you to give it consideration –

From the pen of the truly brilliant functional medicine practitioner, researcher and trainer, Chris Kresser, M.S., LAc,. -

We accept many medical practices and theories without question.

But many of today's most cherished "truths" were viewed as quackery when they were first proposed.

For example, we know with absolute certainty now that bacteria and other germs can cause infection and disease. And we know that using antiseptics and sterilizing equipment during surgery helps to prevent infection and disease.

Yet when Joseph Lister, a surgeon from England, stood before a crowded hall of doctors at Philadelphia's Centennial Exhibition in 1876 and tried to convince them of the importance of antisepsis, he was ridiculed.

Lister knew, without a doubt, that his method was quite literally the difference between life and death. He had conclusive proof from applying antisepsis in surgeries with his own patients and watching the death rate plummet.

But this didn't convince the sceptics.

One doctor said, "The whole theory of antisepsis is not only absurd, it is a positive injury."

Another remarked that Lister's methods "would be a return to the darkest days of ancient surgery."

How could so many medical professionals be so wrong?

In fact, this isn't unusual. The history of medicine is littered with similar examples, from the theory that H. pylori causes ulcers to the discovery of X-rays to the realization that the brain is "plastic" and changes throughout our life.

Despite this, we continue to resist new ideas that are outside of the dominant paradigm.

We make the assumption that although past scientists and doctors were wrong about a lot of things, we've finally got it all figured out.

I would argue that this is anti-scientific, since science relies on our ability to question even our most cherished hypotheses when new evidence comes to light.

Unfortunately, holding on tightly to the status quo

and dominant paradigm seems to be a basic human characteristic, or perhaps a vulnerability.

Perhaps it is related to our strong need to belong socially, which was protective in a natural environment. After all, for our hunter–gatherer ancestors, exclusion from the group (tribe) quite literally meant death.

We're still operating with that same biological programming, but today it shows up in different ways—like not being open to new ideas and new research that contradicts our existing worldview.

It's natural for us to assume that the majority view is always correct.

But history shows us that this isn't a safe assumption.

The French novelist and philosopher Anatole France once said, "Even if 50 million people say a foolish thing, it's still a foolish thing."

Scientific integrity—and progress—demands that we keep our minds open and guard against groupthink, bias, and hubris.

Today's quackery just might be tomorrow's genius.

Whilst I'm not for a minute suggesting that this book's content is 'genius', which it certainly isn't, I have to say that in the world of medical science in general, I totally agree with Chris Kresser.

References

Introduction

Functional medicine–Functional Medicine is a biology-based system that focuses on identifying and addressing the root cause of disease. Visit – www.ifm.org

Chapter Three

Naturopath–A naturopath work with a system of disease treatment that avoids drugs and surgery and emphasizes the use of natural agents. Visit–www.naturopathy.org.uk

Chapter Eight

One radio network – visit–www.oneradionetwork.com

Chapter Nine

Thalidomide was a drug given to pregnant women in the late nineteen-fifties and early nineteen-sixties as a mild sedative. Many patients developed unpleasant side effects, but worse was to come. Many children born to these women had severely deformed limbs.

Chapter Ten

Ayurvedic doctor–Those who practice Ayurvedic medicine believe every person is made of five basic elements found in the universe: space, air, fire, water, and earth, and they treat patients based on that belief.

Visit–www.ayurvedanama.org

Clinical herbalist – A person who practices healing with the use of herbs. Visit – www.associationofmasterherbalists.co.uk

Chapter Eleven

Riverford Organics – visit–www.riverford.co.uk

Abel and Cole–visit – www.abeland cole.co.uk

Chapter Twelve

Berkey filter system – visit – www.berkey-waterfilters.co.uk

Chris Masterjohn – visit – www.chrismasterjohnphd.com

Mike Adams – visit–www.healthranger.com

Chris Wark – visit – www.chrisbeatcancer.com

Chapter Fifteen

Ancient purity–visit – www.ancientpurity.com

Opti MSM – visit – www.amazon.co.uk and enter Opti MSM flakes in the search box.

Evolution organics – www.evolutionorganics.com

Nature's best (for fish oil) – www.naturesbest.co.uk and put maximum omega fish oil I the search box.

Bodykind – visit – www.bodykind.com

Chapter Sixteen

Breathworks – visit–www.breathworks-mindfulness.org.uk

Chapter Eighteen

Superfood world – visit – www.superfood-world.com

Indigo herbs – visit – www.indigo-herbs.co.uk

Chapter Twenty One

Lynne McTaggart – visit – www.wddty.com

Chapter Twenty Two

Bruce Lipton – visit – www.brucelipton.com

Chapter Twenty Four

Claire Weekes – Claire Weekes died in nineteen-ninety aged eighty-seven. Her books and an audio are still available on Amazon.

Glossary of Terms

Allopathic medicine – a system in which medical doctors use drugs and/or surgery to treat the symptoms of disease. More generally called Conventional Medicine.

BRC1/BRC2–human genes that produce tumour suppressor proteins, which can mutate and increase the risk of breast cancer.

COPD – a lung disease characterised by chronic obstruction of lung airflow that interferes with normal breathing.

Diatomaceous earth – the fossilised remains of complex algae (diatoms). Food grade diatomaceous earth is often found in abrasive substances such as toothpaste.

Epigenetics – the study of changes in organisms caused by modification of gene expression rather than the alteration of the genetic code itself.

Glutamate – an important neurotransmitter that plays a role in learning and memory and is vital to the functioning of the brain.

Homeostasis – the process of maintaining a constant internal environment in the body eg a temperature of 37°C. Also used to express 'balance' within the body.

Hubris – excessive pride or self confidence

Hypoglycaemia – a condition where blood sugar levels are below the accepted norms.

Kinesiology – the study of the principles of mechanics and anatomy in relation to human (or non-human) movement

Mindfulness–maintaining a moment-by-moment awareness of thoughts, feelings, bodily sensations, and surrounding environment, through a gentle, nurturing lens–meaning thoughts tune into what we're sensing in the present moment rather than rehashing the past or imagining the future.

Mitochondria – the parts of cells that turns sugars, fats and proteins we eat into forms of chemical energy that the body needs via production of ATP.

Modalities – the method used to treat a patient for a particular condition

Naturopath–a system of treatment of disease that avoids drugs and surgery and emphasizes the use of natural agents (such as air, water, and herbs) and physical means (such as tissue manipulation and electrotherapy)

Neurotoxin–a poison which acts on the nervous system

Nocebo–a detrimental effect on health produced by psychological or psychosomatic factors such as negative expectations of treatment or prognosis.

Parasympathetic nervous system–sometimes called the rest and digest system, the parasympathetic system conserves energy as it slows the heart rate, increases intestinal and gland activity, and relaxes sphincter muscles in the gastrointestinal tract.

Placebo–a medicine or procedure prescribed for the psychological benefit to the patient rather than for any physiological effect.

Positive affirmations–positive phrases which you repeat to yourself which describe how you want to be. The repetition meaning the words sink into your subconscious mind and eventually become your reality.

Sympathetic nervous system – a part of the nervous system that serves to accelerate the heart rate, constrict blood vessels, and raise blood pressure. Is responsible for the response commonly referred to as "fight or flight,"

Transdermal application–a route of administration wherein active ingredients are delivered across the skin and into the blood stream for systemic distribution.

FICTION BY ROGER KNOWLES

Bug
Featuring DI Jack Hogg & DS Peter Edwards

Harry Tompkin only leaves his grimy bedsit above a chip shop to go to work. Known since childhood as Smelly Harry, he's not once missed a day at the factory in over forty years, despite the constant derision from his colleagues – after all, where else would he go? Has anyone shown an interest in him, enquired how he is or how he spends the weekend? If they had, he may have told them how much he enjoys woodcarving. But no one ever has, and no one knows or cares that when at home, he skilfully carves intricate mystical creatures from oak, using his one quality possession, his case of specialist wood carving tools.

There is 'life' in Harry's carvings, life that only a craftsman of true genius can create. Hideous caricatures or beautiful works of art? Psychiatrists might argue they are the distorted product of a strange and troubled mind, a mind in turmoil, a mind in pain. But to Harry they are his family, his children. And life with his ever-expanding family could have continued forever. But then he completes his latest work and christens him Toby. As Harry lifts Toby admiringly, Toby sneers and speaks with spine-chilling contempt. "You'll call me by my name, you pathetic fool, you'll call me Bug."

Next morning, reports of mauled domestic pets are reported to council officials. Foxes, they guess. But can foxes open rabbit hutch padlocks? Then a woman's mutilated body is found in a local park. Perhaps an escaped big cat is responsible, or a pack of wild dogs. But forensic examination finds no evidence of animal saliva on the victim.

DI Jack Hogg and DS Peter Edwards are called in to investigate, an investigation that intensifies as each night brings more victims of inhuman depravity.

Meanwhile, back in the bedsit above the chip shop, Harry's family has a new master…Bug.

Broken Cats and Cowboy Hats
Featuring DI Jack Hogg & DS Peter Edwards

To Mark Doughty's dysfunctional family violence was the norm. Once his abusive father was police custody and his mother institutionalised, neighbours praised the authorities for their rescue of baby Mark. The family may have been torn apart by domestic violence, but here was a chance for Mark to heal and mend. He would be safe in the care of the local authority, they assured themselves, looked after and loved, able to learn and grow into a functional member of society, where his past would be firmly behind him.

The reality of being abandoned to an indifferent care system concerned more with paperwork, finances and Ofsted inspections, was somewhat different. Only concerned social worker, Jackie Shannon, attempted to connect with him during his bleak childhood. But an hour's visit once a month, whenever it not cancelled by mandatory training courses, was not enough to prevent Mark from gradually hardening into a man like his father, whose only means of communication was through violence and intimidation.

As he matured the frustration with his dead-end life culminates in a brutal and unprovoked murder.

His arresting officer, DI Jack Hogg, is pleased to see Doughty put away for life. But his worst fears are realised when Mark escapes from custody, obsessed with exacting retribution on the people who he feels are responsible for his situation.

But who does Mark believe is responsible? And is he right?

The Association

The year is 2029. Ben Lake, a phenomenally successful options trader, receives a call from a Lord Godfrey who invites him to what he describes as a seminar.

Initially disinterested, Lake declines the offer but then becomes intrigued when Godfrey talks of immortality and freedom from disease. Out of curiosity, he eventually decides to attend.

What he hears during the seminar horrifies him and he wants nothing to do with Godfrey or what he calls 'The Association'.

He leaves, and people start to die. Ben is then forced into a set of circumstances that he's totally ill-equipped to handle.

To Be a Man

Martin Roberts is his school's rebel without a cause, and all the girls love him. But he has eyes only for one of them–Lisa Godwin. And Lisa Godwin has eyes only for him.

At home, his mother is concerned that Martin has displayed no outward signs of emotion since his father left home. Although he feels it, that lack of outward emotion threatens to spoil the recently established relationship with Lisa.

The only time those emotions – love, rejection, heartbreak–do come to the fore are when they materialise in the songs that he writes as he plays his guitar.

When he leaves school, he and Lisa are forced apart by Lisa's father, and Martin develops an obsession to be a successful songwriter, to give Lisa everything she could ever want and to spend the rest of his life with her.

His obsession slowly creates the fame and fortune that he craves, but what really matters to him, Lisa, is no longer by his side.

Seventeen years later, his mother sits beside his hospital bed, reminiscing on what might have been. She watches her son's lifeforce slowly fade.

To Be a Man is the story of those seventeen years.

Day of Reckoning

Prequel to 'The Naked Emperor'

This prequel to 'The Naked Emperor' is an hour by hour account of the day during which our hapless hero, Simon Jones, realises that his life must change direction if his sanity is to be preserved.

Starting with an accusation of indecent exposure, Simon's day goes from bad to worse and includes incidents involving a pram with a faulty spark plug, a tea break conversation involving death by farts, a spectacle wearing monkey, an exploding boob, a fat man in a bad mood, a chip shop fight, the near purchase of a pet alligator and a carnal interlude ruined by a hind leg.

The Naked Emperor
Sequel to 'Day of Reckoning'

Tired of aggressive, ungrateful customers, especially those inflicted with a micro penis, hapless motor-cycle repair shop owner, Simon Jones, decides that enough is enough. Having created a travesty coffee table, an experience that forced him to dismiss a career in carpentry, he's finally inspired by a newfound 'gift', and decides that it's time to seek a new and better life.

His savvy wife, Hazel, isn't impressed by his 'gift', but agrees that a week's holiday in Cornwall with the kids, Becky and Ben, and their delinquent golden retriever, Orpheus, would be a good idea, a chance to consider their future.

While on the holiday, during which Orpheus steals a picnic prior to a sexual encounter he doesn't welcome, an incident in a gift shop involving a large lady pretending to be an upturned tortoise, sparks an entrepreneurial idea, and they return home full of plans to create a new business. Initially, the business goes very well until an unanticipated disaster related to cosmetics that turn to cardboard strikes, leading to near bankruptcy.

Desperate for money, Simon has a short spell working in a factory warehouse counting washers, followed by a longer one as an unsuccessful insurance salesman.

One day he returns home from work, broke and full of despair, to be met by someone from the past, someone who, with the help of the naked emperor syndrome, eventually leads Simon and Hazel to a new life of fame and fortune.

Printed in Great Britain
by Amazon